# Setting Standards for Professional Nursing:

## The Marker Model

by Carolyn G. Smith-Marker, MSN, RN, CNA

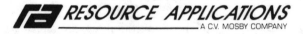

*RESOURCE APPLICATIONS*
A C.V. MOSBY COMPANY

7250 Parkway Drive
Hanover, Maryland 21076
(301) 796-9010
(800) 826-1877

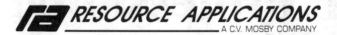
**RESOURCE APPLICATIONS**
A C.V. MOSBY COMPANY

**Resource Applications** is a network of educators and clinicians committed to lifelong learning for health care professionals, and excellence in education.

**Resource Applications** offers:

A comprehensive program of continuing professional education.

An ongoing mechanism for updating clinical competence and professionalism.

A unique approach to education that "bridges the gap" between theory/research and clinical practice.

A unique network of talented clinical and management consultants from across the United States and Canada.

| | |
|---|---|
| Publishing Director | Jay Katz, MA |
| Editorial Director | Jacqueline Katz, MS, RN |
| Editors | Susan Glover, RN, MSN |
| | Jeff Griffith, PhD. |
| Design and Typography | The Graphics Group |

Printed in the United States of America          ISBN 0-8016-5261-8

The C.V. Mosby Company,
11820 Westline Industrial Drive, St. Louis, Missouri  63146

# About the Author

Carolyn Smith-Marker is a Management Specialist with over 20 years of experience. During the past seven years, as a Consultant for Resource Applications, Ms. Marker has concentrated on the development of a framework for writing and implementing Nursing Standards. She is also well known for her work in Quality Assurance.

Each year, thousands of nurses attend her workshops and hundreds of institutions are patterning their standards approaches on her work. Ms. Marker is a dynamic and insightful workshop leader who combines futuristic and pragmatic thinking into a "real world" approach to standards and Quality Assurance.

Carolyn completed her Master's degree in Nursing at Catholic University and her undergraduate degree at Texas Woman's University. She is certified in Nursing Administration by the American Nurses Association.

# Acknowledgements:

As anyone who has attempted to put their thoughts and opinions down in writing knows, successful publication depends on the efforts of numerous persons. I wish to thank the staff of **Resource Applications, Inc.** (past and present), especially Jay Katz, President and Jackie Katz, Vice President, Professional Services, for their assistance and suggestions in the final product, though I know the meeting of great minds is sometimes difficult. A special acknowledgement to Sue Glover for editing my "voluminous verbage" and to all for helping to make a "readable" contribution to nursing literature.

Second, a sincere appreciation to my nursing colleagues who have and are working hard to define our nursing practice through standards and the Marker Model and who have been waiting patiently for this book. I hope it helps! Thank you for your attendance at the seminars, the invitations to your hospitals, and your positive feedback.

Finally, a special thank you to my husband, Chick, who, as many of you have said to me, "must really be someone special," to give the continuous support and encouragement to me to keep up the pace and enthusiasm needed to move a profession forward. His sense of humor has never failed to make me smile. As I have shared with many of you, his famous words—"You're a pioneer, dear, and pioneers occasionally get shot at!" There are a lot of pioneers out there—may we all be successful in influencing nursing for the better.

Carolyn G. Smith-Marker

# Preface

**Setting Standards of Patient Care** presents a comprehensive Model for the development and implementation of nursing standards—hospital-wide or unit specific. It emphasizes organization, methodology, terminology and style in an attempt to "standardize" the way to write standards.

The book is written for every nurse challenged with the responsibility to develop nursing standards whatever the practice setting. It is beneficial as a guide to developing standards where none exist or as a barometer to measure current standards.

Staff will learn what standards are, why they are needed and how they can participate in the Standards Development Project. Nurse managers will learn how all aspects of their leadership role can be incorporated into standards and how to use standards to improve unit function, staff performance, and patient care. Nurse executives will be able to relate standards to overall department objectives, cost-containment measures, quality assurance activities, and regulatory agency requirements. Faculty will draw implications for utilizing standards to build curricula and ease the transition from student to practitioner.

The material does **not** attempt to define what nursing care should be, rather it provides the tools by which nurses can define it themselves. What constitutes appropriate nursing interventions, staff responsibilities, and systems operations for a particular institution is unique to that institution. The book **does** attempt to define the format and style by which those interventions, responsibilities, and operations are written and organized.

Additionally, the book provides a Model for writing standards for all types of patients in all types of settings. Typically, however, the examples used are medical-surgical in nature.

The book is directed into five units which progress sequentially through the Model, each unit building upon the previous units. **Unit I** introduces you to standards. Chapter 1 discusses nursing standards and their 'raison d'etre'. Chapter 2 provides an overview of the Marker Model as the conceptual framework for standards development.

**Unit II** defines Structure Standards as the foundation of the Standards Development Project. Chapter 3 discusses strategies for Policy development and the content of those Policies. Chapter 4 through 7 address the development of specific Policy statements relative to each of the critical elements defined in Chapter 3.

Process Standards are the focus of **Unit III**.

Chapter 8 differentiates Job Descriptions and Performance Standards. Chapter 9 focuses on how to design comprehensive, useable Procedures and Protocols. In Chapter 10, you learn to write Guidelines that specify how forms are to be completed. Discussion is also directed at Standards of Care. The major difference between Standard Care Plans and Standard Care Statements, when each should be used and how they are developed, are discussed.

**Unit IV** addresses Outcome Standards—how they are used, different types and how to incorporate them into your standards.

**Unit V** pulls it all together. It begins by validating your understanding of and skills applying the Marker Model through a series of exercises in Chapter 12. Chapter 13 covers the pragmatics of actually putting together a Unit Standards Manual. Finally a Sample Unit Standards Manual demonstrates more extensive examples of Structure and Process Standards according to the Marker Model for a typical medical-surgical unit. Although the manual is not meant to be complete, it does include a full set of Structure Standards for a bedded, moderate acuity nursing unit, Performance Standards, a sample Procedure, several sample Protocols demonstrating different levels, a sample set of Guidelines, and samples of two different styles of Standards of Care. Due to the page size of this manual, the page restrictions suggested for Policies, Procedures and Protocols were not adhered to.

In each unit, the text is detailed, complete with operational definitions. A glossary is included for easy reference. Diagrams, charts, and sample forms are included to illustrate technical style. In general, this book is a working reference manual for standards development according to the **Marker Model**. It provides the theory, tools, and methods to propel your unit, department or entire system into the "new wave" of nursing practice.

# From the Author . . .

Those who practice, administrate, and teach nursing have long struggled to define the term using a variety of words, phrases, and paragraphs. It is time to move beyond the mere word, nursing, and focus more comprehensively on defining its realistic practice in today's health care facilities. While there is a wealth of information on nursing care, these books, articles and programs generally reiterate the clinical, scientific, and theoretical basis for care. These compilations constitute one or more authors' interpretations of facts and ideas and serve as our professional references. But references are not standards. There are limited seminars and texts addressing nursing standards but these have failed to provide nursing with the necessary tools to define our practice. The work of defining professional nursing practice through written standards still remains to be done and is the ultimate responsibility of each practitioner in every nursing system.

The issue of nursing standards is a current one and information on the topic will, no doubt, proliferate in a short time. The reader must be alert to the information and selective about the ideas he embraces lest he be led astray. Defining the practice of nursing in writing can, in itself, be overwhelming due to the scope and complexity of our profession and nursing systems. The last thing we need is more confusion, diametrically opposed courses, conflicting terminology, and ambiguous direction to encumber our efforts. What we do need is a consistent methodology by which to develop nursing standards that is applicable to all settings. It is to this end that the **Marker Model** was developed and this book was written.

I believe the book presents to the reader something that does not currently exist in any publication or workshop offering: A comprehensive and systematic approach to defining professional nursing. The approach is comprehensive in addressing the three essential components of practice: the system that facilitates and supports the practice; the staff who give care and the patients who receive it; and the end results. The approach is systematic because it stresses the organized building of standards in a hierarchial fashion beginning with the most important aspects of practice and evolving to the most sophisticated. The book clarifies standards terminology by defining words clearly and consistently. It does not add arbitrary new words but explicitly uses terms familiar to most nurses. It avoids buzz term jargon and reduces confusion in communication among practitioners, facilities, and regulatory agencies. This last issue is particularly important because the lack of consistent standards language continues to bog down many systems in wasted time, energy, and disagreement.

I remind the readers that the Marker Model is original thought, created in the clinical setting and developed into a practical approach for getting a job done. It is still evolving. I think its implications and applications to our profession are great. The more I work with the Model and teach it to others, the more amazed I become at its serendipitous possibilities. It began simply as a way to write nursing standards and can be the basis for all activities, responsibilities, and programs that we value.

So take it for what it is—a system to define what we are, organize our work, and streamline our nursing agencies. Make it work for you—don't be a slave to it. It's flexible; shape it to your values and system but not so far as to break it apart. It will not be easy. Significant and visionary endeavors seldom are! Organizing your nursing units, divisions, and departments through written standards will require education, commitment, hard work, time and indirect dollars. Each one of you has to determine whether it is worth it. You'll be asked to abandon traditional thought and to think beyond the "policy and procedure" boundaries that have limited our definition of our practice to date. Instead, you will be challenged to think of all nursing as structure, process, or outcome and to respond accordingly. You'll have to gear up your "left brain" and approach nursing systematically, breaking it down into its component parts and then putting it back together again in a rational and logical manner. You'll have to exercise your "right brain," too, in order to create definition of practice and care where it does not currently exist. The Model will not fail you—it does provide answers to problems and issues which have impeded us for a long time.

We all are experiencing difficult and changing times as health care professionals. I believe we can emerge from current problems and pressures a stronger profession if we work to define our practice, determine its economic value, and justify our indispensible contribution to the consumer. The Marker Model has been shared with hundreds of nurses and systems and is being implemented in many of them. Our goals for our nursing profession are probably very much the same; let us end our disjointed, fragmented, and haphazard efforts and unite our profession through standards.

# Table of Contents

# UNIT I NURSING STANDARDS:

## The building blocks of professional practice

Nurses can function according to defined purposeful expectations or by intuition. A nursing system can operate in a designated manner or haphazardly. Patient care can be delivered by design or by impulse and habit. Standards either exist or they do not. If they exist, they must be detailed, consistent and comprehensive or they will be shallow, irrelevant, and worthless.

Staff nurses often find themselves working without detailed nursing standards that define what is expected of them. This situation is not only frustrating but can also lead to confusion and error in patient care, and to general bewilderment about how things are to be done and what constitutes acceptable performance.

Certain nursing standards do exist, of course, some quite explicit. Failure to comply with standards developed by governmental agencies, for example, can result in severe penalties, such as the loss of Medicare or Medicaid reimbursement or even hospital accreditation. But the penalties for not meeting most professional standards are far less tangible. Noncompliance can be easily justified. A nursing manager can simply say she doesn't agree with the goals and philosophy of the organization that developed the standards. On the whole, professional nursing standards have become synonymous with superfluous paper work that ultimately keeps good nurses away from the patient's bedside.

It's time for that to change. It's time for us to realize that developing nursing standards is the way to eliminate the confusion, frustration, and skepticism that permeate the modern nursing profession.

Education is the key to making that change. We must familiarize ourselves with nursing standards, with the reason and purpose for their existence, and with the factors involved in developing and using them. If we do this, we will come to see both the inadequacies of practicing nursing without well-defined standards and the rewards that await both nurses and their patients when standards become the focus of professional nursing, the very basis for all nursing actions.

# Chapter 1  Nursing By Definition or Assumption?

## WHAT IS A NURSING STANDARD?

A nursing standard is a written value statement that defines a level of performance (in the staff) or a set of conditions (in the system or the patient) determined to be acceptable by some authority. Putting a standard in writing serves several purposes. First, it formalizes the standard, putting it in black and white, so that one can easily refer to it. Second, written standards that define acceptable levels of performance, patient care, and system operations can serve as a keystone around which other programs, such as orientation, quality assurance, and performance appraisal can be built. Third, written standards provide definition of nursing care and control of obstacles that impede care. The quality of patient care on any nursing unit depends on many factors, including staffing patterns, available equipment, safety, and staff knowledge and skill level. Written standards constitute a serious effort to control these factors. Fourth, written standards delineate professional accountability.

Accountability—there's the rub! Being only human, we all tend to fear strict accountability for our actions. This fear can lead to some cozy rationalizations. Consider these comments:

> STAFF NURSE: *"Who's going to care for the patients while we spend all this time writing standards? We know what good care is; we do it everyday!"* (This is the assumption that everybody knows what good care is).

> PHYSICIAN: *"Standards represent a cookbook approach to care. Medicine, and maybe nursing, are too mysterious and ethereal, and variable to be captured by words on paper. Every situation is so different."*

NURSE MANAGER: *"If I write everything down in a standard, what will happen to professional autonomy, decision making, and independent nursing judgment? Standards will turn my nurses into robots!!"*

ADMINISTRATION: *"Detailed standards make care too specific and may increase the institution's liability for negligence."*

Let's examine each objection:

### *"Takes too much time."*

Yes, standards development requires time and probably will go on for months or years. It is a dynamic process. But in the long run, it will benefit each nurse, each system, and every patient. Well developed standards save time by reducing confusion, duplication, and errors of omission.

### *"Not everything can be defined."*

Maybe not, but have we really tried to define the areas of nursing practice that allow delineation? Is the question "Can nursing practice be defined?" or is the question more appropriately, "Have we found a suitable and comprehensive **way** to define nursing practice?" Also, let us honestly consider whether every patient or situation is really so different. Could it be that every nurse's response, knowledge, and skill level is the variable that is so unpredictable? Some situations may not be possible to standardize but these must be the exception and not the rule.

### *"Standards reduce autonomy and independent nursing judgment."*

Nothing could be further from the truth!! When nurses develop standards participatively, they have the real opportunity to incorporate their judgment and decision making into the content of the standards. Standards may contain as much independent nursing function as the institution and law allow. In the daily use of nursing standards, every professional nurse has the right and the obligation to individualize every standard to each patient. Failing to do so would indeed be negligence! Standards do not reduce nursing autonomy, they maximize it. Standards simply define patient care and nursing functions and prevent everyone from doing their "own thing."

### *"Detailed standards increase liability."*

Another fallacy! Much malpractice today involves lack of defined standards which, if in operation, probably would have protected the patient, staff, and facility. The presence of standards is not what we must fear; their absence makes us vulnerable! A lack of detail could communicate an acceptance of superficial care and staff function. The presence of well developed standards and their consistent application are major factors in risk management. Professionals and health care facilities will always be held accountable. The question is "Do you or do you not want to know precisely to which standards you will be held accountable?"

# WHO NEEDS MORE STANDARDS?

This is perhaps the coziest rationalization of all. With so many standards already in existence, who needs more? Don't these existing standards adequately define the practice of nurses, regardless of their institutions and functions, whether clinical or managerial? **Legal standards,** such as the Nurse Practice Act, define the practice of professional nursing within your state. **Professional standards** have been developed by nursing organizations, such as the American Nurses Association (ANA) the American Association of Critical Care Nurses (AACN), the Emergency Nurses Association (ENA), and the Association of Operating Room Nurses (AORN). **Regulatory standards** are drawn up by your local and state health departments and the Joint Commission for the Accreditation of Hospitals (JCAH) for purposes of licensing and accreditation.

If you familiarize yourself with the existing standards, you'll find that many are phrased in general terms. For example, both the ANA and AACN base their standards on the Nursing Process. The content defining the use of assessment, nursing diagnosis, planning, intervention, and evaluation is broadly written so that it can apply to different situations in various practice settings. Each particular nursing unit must review these existing standards and determine their applicability to that unit, its patient population, and staff. Thus, each unit would need to select appropriate assessment data for a patient population and create a Nursing Data Base with guidelines to define its use. Each unit would determine the staff's specific use of nursing diagnosis for incorporation into performance standards. Each unit would define specific interventions to be carried out on its patient populations as well as outcomes to be achieved and then incorporate these into standards of care and associated protocols. Existing standards provide a broad base of function, but must extend into more specific unit, division, and department standards by which to provide care.

# WHAT IS THE LANGUAGE OF CLOUT?

Not all existing standards are mandatory. **Mandatory standards** leave no room for choice. They dictate both the end to be achieved and the means by which it is to be achieved. Examples would be any legal or regulatory standards, such as state health laws, the nurse practice act, and most JCAH requirements, which, if violated, can result in loss of accreditation. These mandatory standards can be recognized by the use of the verbs **shall, will,** and **must**—the language of clout. More recently in regulatory agency literature, these words are eliminated and the present tense is used as "is" or "are" to make a statement of fact about what indeed is mandated. **Voluntary suggestions** state a preference for a particular means of accomplishing some end, without making it mandatory. Alternate means of reaching the same end may be accepted. These standards can be recognized by the use of the verb **should. Voluntary recommendations** are suggestions without even an implied preference. Both the end and the means are optional. These standards can be recognized by the phrase **"It is recommended that. . ."** or the use of the verb **may.** Being aware of the different ways to state a standard is important. You want your intent to be clear. The language of standards is significant when you write your standards and when you interpret those written by others.

### Standards And JCAH

The accreditation manuals published annually by the JCAH identify those structural characteristics required for survey and accreditation in your facility. An important part of preparing for an accreditation and rating well with the surveyors is being very familiar with the accreditation standards. While it is appropriate to be aware of standards that impact on the Nursing Department such as pharmacy, pulmonary function, medical records, medical staff, quality assurance, and infection control, it is imperative to be intimately knowledgeable about the Nursing Service requirements themselves. Consider the Nursing Service Standards VII in the 1987 *JCAH Accreditation Manual for Hospitals:*

Standard

12.7     Written policies and procedures that reflect optimal standards of nursing practice guide the provisions of nursing care.

Required Characteristics

1 2 . 7 . 1 Written standards of nursing practice and related policies and procedures define and describe the scope and conduct of patient care provided by the nursing staff.

These statements require nursing departments to write specific standards defining nursing responsibilities, systems function, and the quality of patient care to be provided. They do not, however, dictate the precise content of those standards, nor the manner in which they are to be written, except to state that they must be related to at least the following ten areas:

- Assignment of nursing care consistent with patient needs, as determined by the nursing process;
- Acknowledgement, coordination, and implementation of diagnostic and therapeutic orders of medical staff members;
- Medication administration;
- Confidentiality of information;
- The role of nursing staff in discharge planning;
- The role of nursing staff in patient/family education;
- Maintenance of required records, reports, and statistical information;
- Cardiopulmonary resuscitation;
- Patient, employee, and visitor safety; and
- The scope of activity of volunteers or paid attendants.

The actual content of the standards that relate to each of these areas remains the prerogative of each nursing department. JCAH establishes "the bottom line;" you take it from there.

# WHY STANDARDS NOW?

Developing lucid nursing standards is a particularly timely concern now because of the advent of Diagnosis Related Groups (DRG's).

Over the past two decades, health care costs have escalated disproportionately compared to the rest of the economy. To control expenditures, the federal government started a prospective reimbursement plan that is based on the patient's diagnosis and the projected length of hospitalization. Under this plan, hospitals receive a predetermined amount of money to cover the cost of caring for Medicare patients. The plan uses economic incentives to motivate hospitals to control costs. If a hospital provides care at a cost below the predetermined allotment, it keeps the difference. If the cost exceeds the allotment, the hospital sustains a loss.

Because DRG's may be here to stay, nursing departments must now control costs, eliminating all wasteful expenditures, while continuing to insure effective patient care. The most rational way to care for sick people under such economic restraints is to define competent professional care as precisely as possible. Given finite dollars, time, and people with which to do the job, the guesswork must be removed from nursing care and replaced with well-defined standards. By delineating roles and responsibilities, by defining who does what, when, where, and how, nurses can begin to control the many tasks that take up our time and energy—and cost money. Such factors as bed utilization; specific admission, transfer, and discharge criteria; equipment; and supplies must be controlled, too.

Most important, the nursing profession must realize that it can benefit from DRG's. Faced with the challenge of cost containment, nursing departments will have to start asking some tough questions. Do all patients require the same level of care? Do all nurses perform basically the same functions? Is the patient's daily room charge appropriate remuneration for bed, board, and the professional nursing services he receives? Administrators will have to explore ways to determine the cost of nursing services so that patients will be charged fairly and the nursing department can receive its rightful share of hospital revenue. Meeting this challenge will not be easy. But by meeting it squarely, by finding the answers to these difficult questions, the profession will grow in knowledge and power. While many efforts at costing out nursing care are being directed at acuity only, a system that has well written nursing standards has an excellent mechanism for correlating cost of nursing care with actual nursing practice. Indeed, the standards themselves can be used as a basis for determining patient acuity and both the quality and quantity of nursing care required by each patient.

# WHAT DO STANDARDS DO?

Standards are a major tool you can use to help you fulfill your role as a nurse manager, to achieve continuous and quality patient care, to insure quality assurance, to improve staff performance, to plan for change, and to solve the problems you face.

## Fulfilling Your Managerial Role

If you ask what a nurse manager does, one might respond by saying nurse managers prepare budgets, conduct evaluations, fill out time schedules and so on. Note, however, that these are **tasks,** and listing the tasks of a nurse manager is like describing the role of the staff nurse by the tasks she performs—hanging IVs, giving medications, changing dressings. The true role of the staff nurse is to carry out the Nursing Process—assessment, nursing diagnosis, goal setting, care planning, implementation and evaluation. The staff nurse performs such tasks as hanging IVs, giving medications, and changing dressings.

The same thing applies to the nurse manager. The true role of the nurse manager is three fold:

To ensure the most efficient unit;
To ensure the most proficient staff; and
To ensure a safe, effective, and appropriate level of care.

In fulfilling this role, the nurse manager, like the staff nurse, performs different tasks. But these tasks should not obscure her broader responsibilities. Developing, implementing, and constantly evaluating standards is the most logical way for the nurse manager to fulfill her true role. This is because standards address all three of the primary elements in any nursing environment—the nurse herself, the system in which she functions, and the patients.

The first responsibility of a nurse manager is to the **system** she operates, whether she supervises a shift, a unit, a division, or an entire department. She must build a system in which professional nursing practice can thrive. No matter how many nurses she has to work with or how well they are educated, they can't give good patient care in a system riddled with chaos, confusion, duplication of effort, outright errors, and too many ways of doing things. Such a system frustrates the staff as well as the managers and jeopardizes patient care. By creating a proficient **staff** that can function in a supportive and consistent system, the nurse manager can meet her third and ultimately most sophisticated responsibility—to the **patient.** These three primary elements serve as the basic building blocks of professional practice—Structure, Process, and Outcome.

Standards can also serve to strengthen any nursing system in five critical management areas:

- Selecting, hiring and retaining nurses;
- Orienting and preparing new nurses;
- Creating a meaningful staff development program;
- Defining a delivery of care system; and
- Conducting meaningful performance appraisals.

Considerable manpower, committee work, time, and energy are required in these areas. Standards are intimately related to each.

Before selecting and hiring new nurses, expectations should be defined through standards so that resume and interview information can be matched with the responsibilities specified. Does the applicant fit your needs? How can you tell if you haven't defined exactly what you need in a nursing staff. Failing to specify responsibilities soon results in the hiring of "warm bodies" who are unprepared for the challenges they will face. Eventually, disappointment for both the employee and employer, high turnover rates among the nursing staff because of frustration over a lack of power in patient care issues, and feelings of disrespect and even apathy toward management and the medical staff result. Developing standards can counteract these negative factors that contribute to low morale. By giving all nurses a voice in defining patient care, standards can produce a sense of pride and accomplishment instead of bitterness and discontent.

You know how valuable orientation programs are, but how many nurse managers are satisfied with the results of these programs? The problem may stem from placing the "orientation cart" before the "standards horse," if you will. An orientation program is designed to help new nurses adjust to new ways of doing things. Building such a program around written standards eliminates the confusion of different preceptors telling orientees different ways of doing the same thing, contributing to inconsistent performance. Your orientation program will succeed—regardless of its design, length, or the use of preceptors—if it is based on well-defined standards related to unit operation, staff performance, and patient care.

No one doubts the validity of creating a staff development program aimed at keeping nurses up-to-date on the latest innovations and creating new areas of expertise. But every staff development session should include a review of standards pertaining to the subject under discussion—either existing standards or standards that need to be developed. Of what practical use is it for nurses to review the anatomy and physiology of the neurological system if they can't relate it precisely to what is expected of them during a neurological assessment? Why educate a nursing staff about the pathology of AIDS if it doesn't result in Standards of Care that incorporate this information in a meaningful way? Why discuss the signs and symptoms of a grand mal seizure, a blood transfusion reaction, or hypovolemic shock unless it can be translated into specific protocols for nursing intervention? Clearly, the linking of staff development programs to nursing standards can strengthen any system's continuing education efforts.

Defining a delivery of care system can benefit from standards. No delivery of care system, whether primary nursing, team or modular, can achieve a consistently high level of staff performance without detailed standards that define exactly what "high level" means. If standards come first, then almost any well-conceived and realistic delivery of care system is possible to implement.

Finally, performance appraisals must proceed on the basis of standards for the position held by the nurse being evaluated. Job descriptions are woefully inadequate for this purpose. They tend to be too vague, too general, and sometimes misleading, not at all reflecting the actual tasks the jobholder winds up performing in the real day-to-day world. Performance Standards sharpen the focus of evaluations by defining beforehand exactly what is expected of the nurse in relation to her knowledge and level of skill. Moreover, her responses to specific patient situations can be more accurately assessed if standards have been developed to cover such situations.

## Achieving Continuous And Consistent Quality Patient Care

Do any of the following situations sound familiar?

- You make rounds and the patient care you see being delivered by your staff doesn't please you.
- You pick up a chart and the quality of documentation does not present an accurate picture of the patient's progress or nursing care delivered.
- You get consistent complaints from the nursing staff that "certain" physicians have not been seeing their patients on a timely basis and that medical orders are too vague and difficult to read.
- Your nursing care plans suffer from the "Blank Kardex Syndrome."
- You go to the central supply cart and note that stock items you need to run your unit are missing, misplaced, or mislabeled.

These situations typify the kinds of problems that you face every day in your unit or division. Such problems represent obstacles that stand in the way of quality nursing care, obstacles that can be removed through standards.

*Consider this:* Maintaining skin integrity is essential to quality nursing care. If less than one percent of the patients on Eight West develop decubitus ulcers during their hospitalization, does that mean the quality of nursing care there is better than that given on Seven East, where five percent of the patients develop decubitus ulcers?

Sensing the statistical trap immediately, you ask yourself: Are there differences in the patient populations of these two units? Are the patients on Seven East immobilized, elderly, debilitated, or malnourished, while those on Eight West are young, ambulatory, elective surgery patients? Such reasoning demonstrates your intuitive understanding of a fundamental fact—that quality nursing care is relative. Conceivably, both Seven East and Eight West could be delivering quality nursing care and achieving those statistics, given the differences in patient populations just described.

But if you were the nurse manager of Seven East and you felt that the five percent decubitus ulcer incidence among your patients could be reduced, what measures would you take? Your staff already knows that frequent skin inspection, turning, repositioning, skin care, and protective devices like sheepskins help maintain skin integrity. But are these measures written down anywhere, spelling out exactly what is to be done, when, by whom, and how the results are to be evaluated? Are they written down on the Kardex? In the patient's chart? In the procedure book? More likely, they are assumed to be in every nurse's head. How do you know they're being carried out? Would you and your staff be able to prove that, despite your very best efforts at maintaining skin integrity, a few severely debilitated, cachectic, and malnourished patients will inexorably suffer skin breakdown? Standards—and frequent evaluations of staff compliance to standards—can provide such proof.

What about continuity and consistency? Quality nursing care, everyone agrees, must be both continuous and consistent. Let's look at what these two words mean.

**Continuity** refers to round-the-clock care given from shift to shift, day to day, by the many nurses who interact with a patient.

**Consistency** refers to the same level of care given patients with the same diagnosis. Do all cholecystectomy patients on your unit or even department receive the same level of care? Or does the level of knowledge and skill (and yes, even the mood) of the nurse assigned to one of those cholecystectomy patients affect the level of care that patient will receive on a particular shift?

The variables that can interfere with these high-minded objectives are obvious—nurse/patient ratios, short staffing, different knowledge and skill levels, different degrees of commitment, and a lack of standards.

Nursing has long recognized these problems and attempted to deal with them. Primary nursing care is designed to promote continuity and consistency. But primary nursing, just like team, modular, case, and functional nursing, is only a delivery of care system. We can't ensure that the care a primary nurse plans and directs for her patients will achieve continuity and consistency until we have defined this care and proven that it is being met. Consider these examples:

- Primary Nurse X orders respiratory assessment for each of her cholecystectomy patients performed twice per shift for the first 48 hours post-operatively.

- Night Nurse Y feels that this is excessively disturbing to patients' rest and only carries out respiratory assessment once on her shift.

- Primary Nurse Z orders respiratory assessment for her patients during the first 72 hours post-cholecystectomy—to include chest auscultation for rales, rhonchi, and wheezing, as well as respiratory rate and character—performed at the beginning and middle of each shift by the associate RN. (Her clinical experience and literature search have demonstrated that patients with upper abdominal incisions are at the highest risk of developing atelectasis in the first three days postoperatively).

Which nurse would you rather have caring for you? What does Nurse X mean by respiratory assessment? Shouldn't Nurse X and Z have the same standard for respiratory assessment of post-cholecystectomy patients? How can Night Nurse Y be prevented from doing her own thing? Without standards, none of these issues can be successfully resolved. The patient becomes the victim of "nurse roulette," dependent on the level of knowledge and skill of his assigned nurse, her ability to define his care in objective and specific terms, and ultimately her ability to ensure that the system will follow through on her directives. Unless nursing standards are defined, and a method for ensuring compliance to those standards developed, the patient remains vulnerable to discontinuous and inconsistent care, regardless of the delivery of care system adopted.

What about the care delivered on different units? If you're a middle manager with responsibility for different units, you must be concerned about inter-unit standards. Patients and staff move from unit to unit. Radical differences in the level of care delivered among units is disconcerting to patients and demoralizing to staff. Control the level of care through inter-unit standards that insure continuity and consistency across units within a division.

Finally, if you are a Director or Vice-President of Nursing, you are going to be concerned that all divisions within your department have comparable standards—standards that are consistent with the department's philosophy and the existing policies that govern your institution. Such intra-departmental standardization is a prerequisite for ensuring quality care that is both continuous and consistent throughout the nursing service.

### Insuring Quality Assurance

Writing standards is only a means to an end. The end to be achieved in this case is quality—quality staff performance, systems operations, and patient care. Writing standards can define quality, but only compliance to standards can achieve quality. And only a quality assurance program, a JCAH mandate for nursing departments, can ensure such compliance. A quality assurance program documents compliance or noncompliance with standards. If you are in compliance with standards, you are delivering quality care by your own definition. But if you find noncompliance, you know that you're falling short of your own standards.

Standards are **never** an end in themselves. They are **always** a means to the end. Quality is always the end that must be defined by standards and is accomplished by instituting a quality assurance program (QAP). QAP is a creative system in which you document compliance/noncompliance with standards and thus validate quality care or identify problems which prevent quality.

The two basic approaches to evaluating the quality of patient care are problem-focused and compliance-focused. Certainly you need to establish mechanisms for identifying and reporting problems that negatively affect patient care. But waiting for these problems to arise may invite patient injury, institutional liability, and staff frustration. Isn't it better to anticipate problems through compliance review by actually monitoring compliance or noncompliance with your standards? When compliance drops below a specified level, you've identified a problem that needs to be solved. The compliance-focused approach keeps you on top of things and prevents molehills from becoming mountains.

Ultimately, standards make developing meaningful criteria for evaluating compliance or noncompliance possible—a necessary step before any quality assurance program can be successfully implemented. **Criteria** are reliable indices of quality care which identify the key elements in such care. When criteria are met, compliance to the standards is demonstrated; when they are not met, this reflects noncompliance.

Criteria should be developed only when you reach the evaluation stage. Standards **always** come first: criteria evolve out of them. If an evaluation is conducted in the absence of standards, then the criteria by which performance or care is being judged will be arbitrary and subjective. This is unfair to the staff being evaluated and generally leads to poor results.

## Improving Staff Performance

Standards can be an invaluable tool for improving staff performance. Standards help you educate your staff about quality care, allowing you to define precisely what is expected of them while enlarging their nursing knowledge. Participating in the research and writing of standards is also an educational experience, as is the evaluation of compliance or noncompliance.

Imagine, for example, that you are concerned about your staff's inability to assess and promote the progressive activity of post-myocardial infarction patients. You feel that these patients are immobile for too long, that your nurses lack assertiveness in collaborating with physicians on promoting activity, and that nursing documentation fails to reflect the patients' responses to activity levels. The physicians seem reluctant to progress these patients to higher levels because they don't have faith in the staff's ability to assess negative physiologic effects and to intervene appropriately.

The problem is a lack of both knowledge and clearly defined expectations. It can be solved by researching and writing, in collaboration with the medical staff, a "Protocol for Progressive Activity in the Post-MI Patient." Defining what constitutes the management of progressive activity during the MI healing phase, followed by planned education, active implementation, and quality assurance evaluation activities will produce success. Staff competency and confidence will improve as will patient care.

## Planning For Change

Successful change requires planning. Without planning, the change will be haphazard and ineffective. Volumes have been written on "change theory," but the fundamental principle for changing a nursing system is to plan for change through standards development.

This book discusses three types of standards—Structure, Process, and Outcome—that can successfully initiate a positive change in any nursing department. You will see how you can brainstorm to determine what policies are needed, what new processes are involved, what staff education is necessary, and whether patient outcomes need to be specified. Such intensive analysis will tell you what standards you need to develop to initiate change successfully. Planning for change through standards helps you avoid the pitfalls of chaotic, traumatic change.

Standards facilitate all types of change. Consider the many opportunities for initiating change when creating something new in any nursing environment:

- New units require structure, process, and outcome standards.
- New forms require new guidelines.
- New physicians mean new programs for new patient populations, requiring new procedures, protocols, and standards of care.
- New equipment and products require new procedures and sometimes new protocols.
- New diagnostic and therapeutic modalities require new protocols and often new procedures.
- New expectations for staff require new performance standards.

"New" implies change which requires definition and evaluation through standards.

## Solving Problems

Virtually all nursing problems result from a **lack of standards** or a **lack of compliance to standards.** Ask yourself if you're satisfied with the way you identify and solve problems in your work. Do you really solve problems or do you sometimes feel more like a crisis manager, putting out brushfire after brushfire? Fatigue, frustration, high turnover, recurrent problem issues, complacency, insensitivity, and nonresponsiveness are symptoms of a nursing staff that is not effectively solving problems. They reflect a despairing attitude that problems will always outnumber solutions. But effective problem-solving is possible through standards development. Once you have identified a problem ask yourself, "Do I have a well written standard relative to the problem?" If the answer is no, then the obvious first step toward solving your problem is to develop a standard that addresses the problem. Write a standard that prevents problem occurrence, reduces its frequency, or minimizes its negative impact. Match the type and format of the standard to the issue. Follow these five critical steps:

1. INPUT: Seek input on the standard from all who would be affected by it and those who have the power to institute change. This is the drafting stage where negotiation, collaboration, and communication take place. The final draft emerges from this step.

2. APPROVAL: Obtain approval to give the standard authority. This should include multiple levels of staff, nursing hierarchy, appropriate medical staff, and appropriate committee structure.

3. EDUCATION: Educate those involved on the content and use of the standard. Use post-testing mechanisms to insure that persons responsible for using the standard understand it. Remember that knowledge and commitment go hand-in-hand.

4. IMPLEMENTATION: This is an active process involving role modeling by both managers and staff which maintains staff awareness of the standard. Awareness can be kept at a high level by incorporating new standards into the day-to-day operation of the nursing unit. For example, integrate standards into change of shift reports and weekly patient care conferences. Include some topic of standards at every staff meeting and have one of the staff members review its content and implications for the group. Integrate standards into every staff development session and use new standards as a basis for concurrent monitoring activities in your unit quality assurance program.

5. MONITORING RESULTS: Using quality assurance to follow up the effectiveness of the new standard will not only reflect compliance of the staff to the standard but will also tell you the impact

it has had on the original problem—elimination of the problem, or reduction in its frequency or negative impact.

You'll notice that this five step approach to problem solving does not direct you to "audit" problems. Auditing is not a problem solving activity but a data collection process. Inappropriate auditing of problems can waste time and actually retard important problem resolution. Why waste time auditing problems for which you have no standards? That's just delaying the inevitable! Instead, solve the problem by developing a standard, follow through with implementation, and then demonstrate effectiveness through QA measures.

But suppose you answer, "Yes, I do have a standard." Why would you still have a problem when the standard was designed to prevent it? Obviously, the answer is noncompliance and you have to make an effort to find out who is responsible for the noncompliance. It could be anyone—a staff nurse, a doctor, a nursing supervisor, or the medical director. You also need to determine why someone failed to comply with the written standard so the situation can be corrected. Basically, only three honest reasons for noncompliance exist: "I didn't know how"; "I didn't know I was supposed to"; or "I didn't care."

Ultimately, you will have to be the judge of what is an acceptable justification for not complying with a standard and what is merely an excuse. But if you begin to accept too many excuses—Too busy, Short-staffed, Never got around to it, Someone called in sick—you'll soon find noncompliance on the rise and compliance rapidly declining, along with quality of care! Figure 1-1, depicts the process of problem solving with standards.

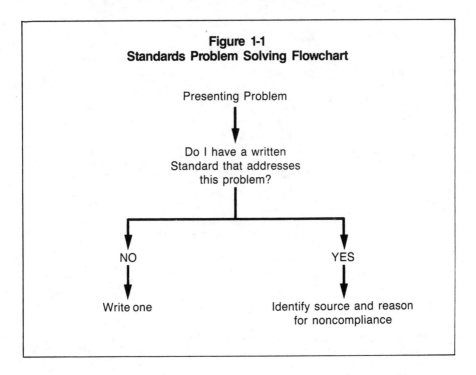

**Figure 1-1**
**Standards Problem Solving Flowchart**

Presenting Problem

Do I have a written
Standard that addresses
this problem?

NO

Write one

YES

Identify source and reason
for noncompliance

Problem-solving, in the end, is the most important of the many functions of standards. It is really what standards are all about. We know there are problems out there that need to be solved in the real world of nursing. Developing nursing standards, thoughtfully conceived, clearly stated, tempered with reality, is the first step toward solving them.

# Chapter 2  The Marker Model—A Hierarchy of Nursing Standards

This chapter is the crux of standards development. We're between two points right now—accepting the challenge of writing standards, as discussed in Chapter 1, and organizing a Standards Development Project. This chapter bridges the gap between the rationale for creating standards and actually preparing to write them. It provides a conceptual framework for standards development.

The Marker Model is graphically depicted as a pyramid. Standards development is the process of building that three dimensional structure.

Side one of the pyramid concerns the three types of standards—**Structure, Process,** and **Outcome**. The Marker Model organizes these three types of standards in a hierarchy—an orderly, graded series arrangement. Not all standards are alike in consequence or complexity. Once standards have been approved, they are all equally powerful. However, some standards are foundational, while others are more sophisticated.

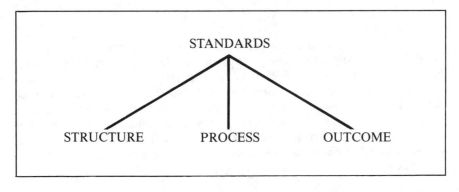

Structure standards provide the solid foundation. Once this foundation has been laid, the second level - (Process) - can be developed. With Structure and Process firmly in place, the apex of the pyramid - (Outcome) - can be appropriately placed. (Figure 2-1)

**Figure 2-1**

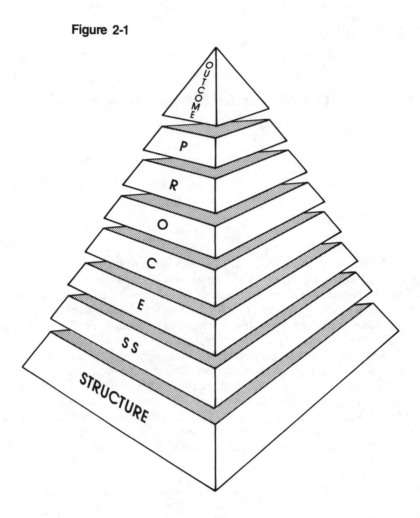

Side two addresses the various formats the three types may take. Standards development consists of matching a topic or issue to a TYPE OF STANDARD and then to the appropriate FORMAT. *Format* reflects the "form" the standard type will take on paper. There are many different formats and these too may be hierarchial in relationship. For example, within process standards, some formats are fundamental while others are more complex. We must continue the hierarchial "brick laying" in a logical order. We'll see how this second level can be directed at either the behaviors of the staff member or the care given the patient.

Figure 2-2 illustrates the relationship of the type of standard and the various formats it may take.

**Figure 2-2**

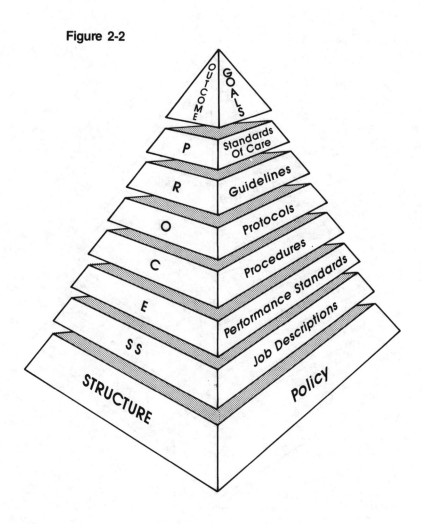

The third side of the pyramid is the quality assurance component, a critical element of each type and format of standards. Figure 2-3 illustrates the relationship of QA to the various Structure, Process and Outcome formats.

**Figure 2-3**

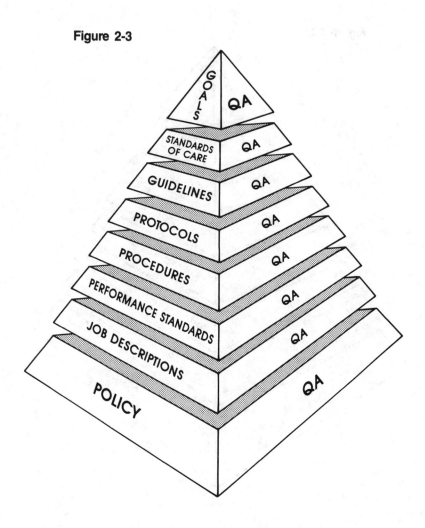

# STRUCTURE STANDARDS—THE FORMAT OF POLICY

*Structure standards define all the conditions and mechanisms needed to operate a nursing system.* As the foundation from which all other standards arise, they address many elements from physical and environmental issues to philosophical and administrative issues. They encompass all aspects of a nursing system except the process of giving care and its desired outcome. Structure standards are written in the format of **POLICY**.

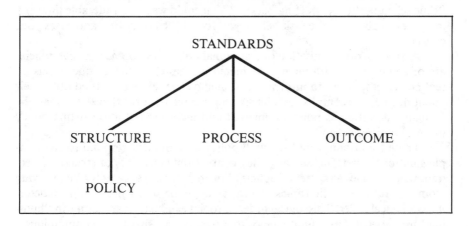

Structure standards must exist at all levels of systems functioning:

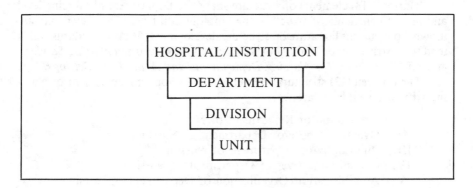

Most institutions have general policies for operation. Each department in turn has more specific policies to address internal concerns. Each nursing department, each division (or cluster of like units), and maybe even each unit should have a set of structure standards to outline its function and operation. Deciding whether to develop structure at the division or unit level will be discussed later in the book. Traditionally, policy content has been poorly defined and, as a result, many topics which are really process issues have been forced into policy. Typically, policies are randomly developed as isolated statements on separate pieces of paper or are combined with procedures and organized alphabetically.

Because a topic can easily be alphabetized under several categories, it is often duplicated under all possible categories. This duplication requires extensive cross referencing and adds more volume. The effect is a massive collection of paper, the traditional policy/procedure manual, which is usually too awkward and time consuming for the average staff nurse or manager to use. An excessive volume of policy statements creates a problem of organization.

Say, for example, you were looking for a nursing policy on floating personnel. Would you look under "floating", "temporary reassignment of staff", "time schedules", or "staffing issues"? You could waste considerable time and maybe even abandon the task before you found the policy that addresses your concern.

Another serious limitation of traditional policy development is that policies are often confused with memos. A memo is simply a communique; it has no real power other than to inform. Most memos should be discarded after their intent has been accomplished. Permanent change requires that the content be formally identified as policy, approved and incorporated into existing policy in an organized manner.

These traditional problems with policy development respond to five simple solutions. First, include as policy content only elements of structure. Second, write policies as a "set of policies" in an outline, paragraph style, flowing from general to specific topics. Third, arrange the set of policies in predetermined, logical order. This logical order of topics eliminates wasted time in "hunting" for issues. Fourth, limit memos to information—sharing of communiques. Fifth, never just "add" new policy on top of old; instead, integrate new into existing Structure.

Thirteen (13) elements of structure shape the Department of Nursing level and nine (9) elements of structure the unit/division level. These elements are drawn from current literature on structure development, JCAH standards which tend to be structure focused, ANA's *Standards for Organized Nursing Services*, and NLN's *Criteria for Nursing Departments and Acute Care Settings*.

The thirteen (13) structural elements for developing Department of Nursing structure standards are:

I. Description of Department of Nursing;
II. Overall Purpose of Department of Nursing;
III. Philosophy of Department of Nursing;
IV. Overall Objectives of Department of Nursing;
V. Administration/Organization of Department of Nursing;
VI. Hours of Operation of Department of Nursing;
VII. Utilization of Patient Care Areas;
VIII. Utilization of Nursing Staff/Staffing;
IX. Maintenance of a Professional Practice System;
X. Governing Rules for Department of Nursing;
XI. Selection/Orientation/Development/Evaluation/Credentialing of Nursing Personnel;
XII. Quality Assurance Activities within Department of Nursing;
XIII. Nursing Responsibilities (generically stated).

The nine (9) structural elements for developing unit/division structure standards are:

I. Description of Nursing unit/division;
II. Overall Purpose of unit/division;
III. Overall Objectives of unit/division;
IV. Administration/Organization of unit/division;
V. Hours of Operation of unit/division;
VI. Utilization of the area (admission, duration of stay, transfer, discharge criteria and planning);
VII. Governing Rules of the unit/division;
VIII. Staffing of the unit/division;
IX. Nursing Responsibilities of the unit/division (specifically stated).

Each element is composed of several components around which the policy statements are developed. Both sets of policies, logically written and organized, enhance each other. No duplication of content occurs. Most importantly, they serve as a ready reference for staff and managers to use in daily decision making.

Structure standards form the base of our Standards pyramid (Figure 2-4). They are the most important type of written standard: more sophisticated Process and Outcome standards evolve from them.

**Figure 2-4**

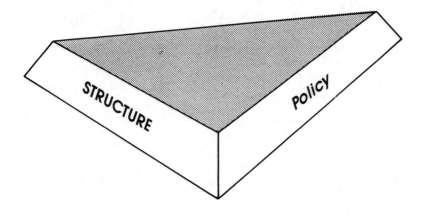

## PROCESS STANDARDS—MULTIPLE FORMATS

Process standards define the actions, knowledge, and skills needed by staff and managers in giving care and also what constitutes that care. These standards make up the bulk of any system's standards project. They can be directed at the nurse or the patient, and because they cover the full range of nursing activities and patient care, Process standards can be cast into six (6) formats:

- Job descriptions,
- Performance standards,
- Procedures,
- Protocols,
- Guidelines,
- Standards of care.

Before we explore the Process formats, let's diagram our discussion to this point:

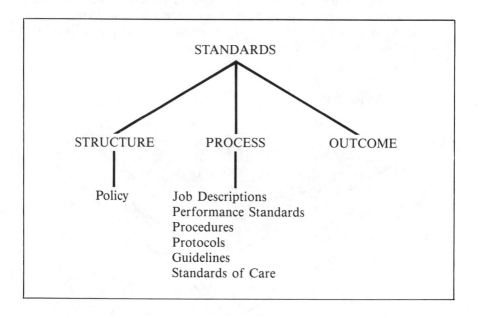

As we review the Process formats, remember the hierarchy. We began with the most important type of standards, Structure. Now we proceed to more complex standards, Process. Each Process format becomes more sophisticated as we climb the standards pyramid. (Figure 2-5).

**Figure 2-5**

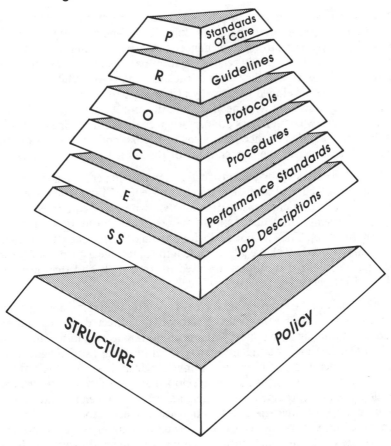

Now, let's look more closely at each of the Process formats.

*Job Descriptions* outline the duties, responsibilities, and qualifications for a level of employee. They are not absolutely specific but provide a realistic overview of what the position entails. The job description is directed at a level or category of worker such as staff RN, head nurse, assistant director, and so forth. Content for developing job descriptions in nursing usually comes from existing standards—legal (Nurse Practice Acts), professional (ANA), and regulatory (JCAH). While the job description is a valuable tool for defining broad requirements of nurse behavior, it does not define precise performance expectations required of nurses working in different areas of MCH, Critical Care, or Medical-

Surgical Nursing. This lack of specificity limits its use as a staff development mechanism and meaningful performance appraisal tool. A clearly written job description simply provides a basis for further development of standards.

*Performance Standards*, on the other hand, are written statements that define specific expectations of behavior, knowledge, and skill required to maintain quality of patient care. Performance standards are extensions of the job description. They are written in relation to three parameters: the patient population, their acuity level, and the values of the nurse manager. While performance standards can be developed generically at the department of nursing level, it is imperative to develop them specifically at the unit level. Thus, while the job description states what all nurses do, performance standards define what specific behaviors are required to meet the needs of the patient population on a particular unit and satisfy the expectations of that unit leader.

*Procedures* are step-by-step instructions on how to perform a psychomotor skill, based on technical and theoretical knowledge. This format limits itself to the details of a particular task, often involving the use of equipment, medication, or treatment. Procedures should be restricted to one or four pages of technical direction. They do not deal with ongoing nursing care. In many nursing systems, procedures have grown in length to become a "catch-all" for inappropriate content. Procedures are used to train skills and then become an occasional reference for review.

*Protocols* are the appropriate format for defining nursing management of broad patient problems or issues. Protocols are directed at managing five categories of nursing care issues: patients on non-invasive equipment; patients with invasive lines and equipment; management of therapeutic, diagnostic, and prophylactic measures; common pathophysiologic and psychologic states; and nursing diagnoses. Protocols may be developed on three different levels: **dependent** (delegated care, requiring a physician's order), **independent** (autonomous nursing action), and **interdependent** (both delegated and autonomous functions). Protocols contain more sophisticated information than procedures and involve extensive use of the nursing process. Protocols define and direct nursing care and will be implemented at the patient's bedside. The protocol may become part of the permanent medical record.

*Guidelines* specify directions for filling out various forms designed for effective communication and documentation, such as data bases, flow sheets, patient progress records, and so forth. Every form used by nurses should have a set of guidelines to insure its proper use.

*Standards of Care* are pre-written plans of care developed for groups of patients about whom generalizations and predictions can be made because they share common problems and needs. Standards of care are different from other Process formats because they are directed toward patients who fit into diagnostic categories—for example, myocardial infarction patients; gastrectomy patients; multiple trauma patients; patients with diabetes mellitus, hypertension, or congestive heart failure, and so forth. These groups of patients can be identified by medical diagnosis or DRG's. In developing Standards of Care for your most common patient populations, you would define the priority nursing diagnoses associated with that DRG, the desired outcomes to be achieved, and the nursing interventions for accomplishing the specific outcomes. Standards of care may be written in two different styles—the traditional **standard care plan** or the newer **standard care statements**. In either approach planning nursing care for groups of patients through standards of care represents the most sophisticated level of process standard that you can write. The Marker Model operationalizes standards of care, like protocols, at the patient's bedside; they may become part of the permanent medical record.

Process standards can be directed at the nurse or the patient. Obviously, job descriptions and performance standards are directed at the nurse, as are procedures and guidelines. But protocols and standards of care are directed at the patient because they spell out the details of patient care, the former outlining broad patient care problems and issues, and the latter dealing with specific patient population groups.

Protocols and standards of care are used to supplement one another. For example, if you were assigned to a patient with a medical diagnosis of upper GI bleeding, post-op hemigastrectomy, the applicable standard of care would be the "Standard of Care for Post-Op Hemigastrectomy Patients". This would address the six priority nursing diagnoses common to that patient population, the desired results, and nursing interventions to be implemented. The standard plan of care would direct you to implement the protocols which would be applicable to this patient's care, i.e. "Post-Op Protocol", "GI Intubation Protocol", "IV Therapy Protocol", and so forth. Thus Standards of Care and Protocols are integrated so that content is not duplicated. This integration saves a great deal of paper and time in the care planning process. Of course various procedures would be performed and guidelines would apply to the relevant documentation forms. This interlocking of Process standards enables you to give care based on all your patient's needs while maximizing the use of nursing resources.

Process standards are the next level in the hierarchy that define your nursing practice and link the system (Structure) with the result (Outcome).

## OUTCOME STANDARDS—STATING YOUR RESULTS

Outcome standards specify the results to be achieved. They are written in the format of a **goal**. Our diagram is complete with the three types and various formats of standards development:

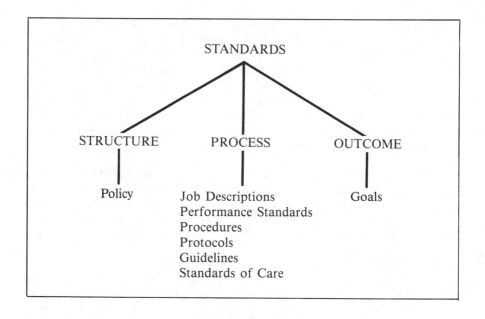

STANDARDS

STRUCTURE          PROCESS          OUTCOME

Policy        Job Descriptions          Goals
              Performance Standards
              Procedures
              Protocols
              Guidelines
              Standards of Care

This third and final type of standard is incorporated into the standards of care for the major patient populations on a nursing unit and into "Teaching Protocols." The Outcome standards link the nursing diagnoses in the standards of care to the specific nursing interventions. They provide direction for the plan and serve as a basis for patient discharge planning as well as outcome review in unit quality assurance activities. Teaching protocols specify the teaching goals and content for patient education. Outcome standards never exist alone, but are part of process standards, specifically, standards of care, and teaching protocols—where they may take two different points of view. Outcome standards may be directed at the nurse as **nursing goals** or they may be directed at the patient as **patient outcomes**. Nursing goals specify what the nurse desires to accomplish as a result of care given. They begin with action verbs. For example, "Prevent post-op atelectasis", "Maintain full ROM in affected extremity", "Minimize further tissue loss at wound site" are outcome standards written as nursing goals. On the other hand, goals written as patient outcomes are statements of condition to be achieved in or by the patient in physiologic, psychologic, or cognitive domain. For example, "The patient will demonstrate healing at the amputation site", "The patient will display behavior indicating acceptance in relation to living with his chronic disability", or "The patient will state knowledge related to medication, dietary, and ADL activities" are patient outcomes. Standards of Care may include both or opt for the patient outcomes only. Teaching protocols use patient outcomes only. Regardless of the style used, Outcome standards are essential to the care planning process and pave the way to effective quality assurance functions. Outcome is the peak of our pyramid. (Figure 2-6).

**Figure 2-6**

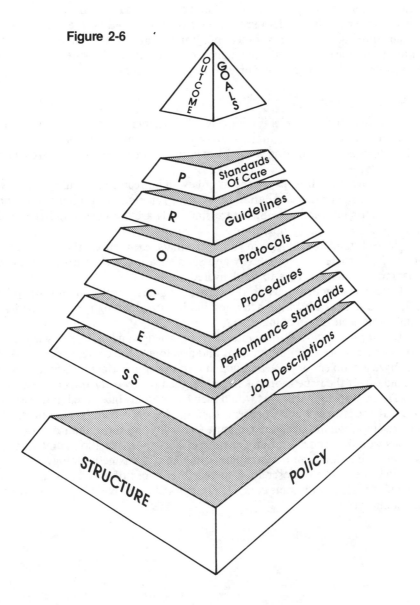

## QUALITY ASSURANCE: THE CRITICAL COMPONENT

The Marker Model reflects our past discussion of the relationship of standards development to quality assurance. The model shows that some aspect of quality assurance should take place consistently along the way as standards are developed. This will assure that the standards are realistic in content and application. Taking time to monitor compliance to standards will help maintain a reasonable pace of development and assure a lasting change. Also, after standards are in place, the model reminds us that they should be the major focus of our nursing quality assurance program. Only when our QA efforts demonstrate consistently high compliance to our standards do patients and nursing staff reap the benefits of our efforts.

## Summary

Now the Marker Model is complete. The schema we have seen evolve can be used to define a nursing unit, a division, or a department. No attempt at defining professional nursing is complete until all three types of standards have been addressed.

Structure standards, expressed as **policy** and directed at defining the nursing system, provide the foundation for systems function, decision making, and all other nursing standards. Structure standards are the most important and establish a solid base of operation.

Process standards, written in various formats, each representing an ascending level of progressive complexity and sophistication, define expected nurse behaviors and patient care to be delivered.

Outcome standards, cast in the format of **goals**, specify the results to be achieved in patient education activities and in care planning for major patient populations seen in a nursing area.

Developing standards demands both knowledge and skill: Knowledge of what nursing issues require standards and developing the content therein; skill to analyze a problem or issue and match it to the appropriate type and format of standard. If the issue is one of structure, then policy is the only correct format. The new policy statements would then be smoothly integrated into existing policy. If the issue is one of process, then the format would be chosen which most easily accommodates the content. Generally, no more than one or two formats would be chosen for any one topic. This approach allows any nursing issue to be developed into a standard using consistent methodology.

Now, let's take a closer look at the three types of standards and their development along with some concrete examples of each. We'll begin with structure standards.

# UNIT II STRUCTURE STANDARDS:

### Building the foundation through policy

No manager can escape the responsibility of formulating and shaping policy. Policy defines and governs the operation of your area, be it a unit, a division, or an entire department. In the Marker Model, policy is the very foundation of your standards system because it helps you weather the storms that strike any busy, dynamic nursing system.

**Structure standards define the conditions and mechanisms needed to operate and control the nursing system**. They are "thing oriented" and written in policy format covering the predefined elements of structure. Structure standards accomplish several purposes: they constitute the base of operation of your area and support your clinical and managerial decision making, they promote the development of more sophisticated standards, and they serve to hold health care members accountable. Structure standards also provide the basis for negotiating and resolving conflict between various disciplines and provide a power base for the practice of nursing. Keep in mind that we are not talking about nursing policies, nor are we referring to medical staff policies. What you will be developing are system policies. At some point these policies will focus strictly on the nurse, at other points your policies will address the physician, and at still other points the focus will be primarily on the system.

# Chapter 3 Introduction to Nursing Policy Development

## DEVELOPING A POWER BASE

Using Structure standards to develop a base of power for clinical and managerial nursing practice cannot be overemphasized. In nursing systems, the units that have grown most rapidly over the last two decades—the units that demand the most staff, the highest percentage of continuing education funds, the largest capital equipment expenditures—are the critical care units. Why? Acuity of patient population, of course, but there's more to it than that. These units have thrived because they have a base of power created by three essential components: 1) solidly developed structure standards in the form of unit policies 2) formalized nurse-physician relationships in the form of appointed medical directors and 3) nurse-physician liaison committees in the form of regularly held meetings where multi-disciplinary problem solving takes place. For years JCAH has directed that critical care areas put these components in place and they have been successful in assisting these areas to function effectively.

But no such direction exists for other units outside the critical care areas such as medical-surgical, psychiatry (acute inpatient units), labor and delivery, post partum, newborn nursery, and the pediatric unit. The lack of these essential components of a power base has created an enormous power gap between these two groups of units, critical care and non-critical care. Therefore, these latter nursing units are often functionally weaker, less organized, and less likely to influence higher level system decision making.

The only way these units can develop a comparable power base is to design their own structure standards to direct operation in their respective areas; to develop organized relationships between medicine and nursing by more clearly defining the roles and responsibilities of physicians including the chiefs of service (i.e. chief of medicine, chief of surgery, chief of orthopaedics, and so forth) to the nurses and the nursing unit; and finally, to organize nurse-physician liaison groups that meet on a regular basis to discuss mutual concerns.

### Levels Of Structure

Structure should exist at all levels of the system. While hospital and department of nursing policies do exist, they are too general to deal with specific concerns of a nursing unit. Structure development must also take place at more fundamental levels of the organization. That's why each nursing unit needs its own structure standards, written as policy, to address its patient population, its unique problems, and the individual nurses and physicians working on that unit.

You may opt for writing Structure standards at the division level where the policies would apply across several units. Since most departments of nursing are broken down into divisions—groups of units with common patient populations and staffs, such as critical care, medical-surgical, psych-mental health, maternal-child health, and so forth—this can be a very workable approach. The choice, however, is between unit and division structure standards because no system needs both. Simply determine which approach best meets your needs.

The decision whether to develop individual unit policy or divisional policy is based on the simple question, "Are you and your sister units more alike or different?" If all units within a division have basically the same patient population, the same staffing requirements with similar responsibilities, and operate in the same manner, you are more alike than different and you need only one set of policies for the division. An example might be six medical-surgical units that share the characteristics listed above. On the other hand, if the units have different patient populations, different staffing requirements with dissimilar responsibilities, and each functions in a unique way, then they are more different than alike. Thus each would require its own set of structure standards. An example would be maternal-child health division where labor and delivery, post partum, newborn nursery, and the pediatric unit would each write their own policies. Of course, they might choose to "link" themselves together via joint objectives and philosophy.

## STRATEGIES FOR DEVELOPING STRUCTURE

Because of the nature of structure standards, physicians, nursing administration, staff, and even hospital administration must be given an opportunity for input and approval of policy. However, nursing management—the head nurse and middle manager—will have the primary responsibility for drafting policy at the unit or division level. This is appropriate because they are the most intimately involved with the day to day operations of the nursing unit and division. Also they usually possess the three requisites for effective policy development: perspective to balance and protect the interests of the system, staff, and patients; systems orientation to understand and relate the complexities of the entire institution to a specific unit or division; and problem solving abilities to continually seek more effective ways of dealing with troublesome issues.

As the most knowledgeable and best prepared to assume this responsibility, the nurse manager must choose a strategy to solicit input from key individuals, most notably physicians, to complete the drafting activities. Often nurse managers and physicians write policies together. If you've ever served on a committee that was responsible for putting something into writing, then you're no doubt familiar with the inevitable hassles over wording. This strategy is best reserved for hammering out areas of disagreement on well defined, isolated issues. Another approach is for nurse managers to write policies and submit them to the medical staff and the hospital administration for input and approval. Nurses do the work but can address issues they feel are appropriate in the way they feel is most effective; then other groups can modify them as necessary. Changing something that already exists is easier than developing something from scratch. So you're more likely to get the feedback you need from physicians if you've given them something with which to work. Submitting your drafted policies for input and approval allows the medical staff to maintain their power base. Most importantly, this strategy is usually the most expedient way to get the job done. This approach is dangerous, however. Certain issues in your unit or division structure will be medically and politically sensitive. If you use this strategy, you must write the content with a sound knowledge of medical staff bylaws and existing administrative policy. For example, if medical staff bylaws state that consultation is strictly the prerogative of the attending physician, you can't presumptuously stipulate in your policies that cardiology consultation is mandatory for all MI patients. If you do, you will have stepped on medical turf, and you can expect to be promptly criticized for your audacity! Don't address such an issue until you've discussed it with the appropriate physicians and negotiated a solution.

Use your knowledge of existing policy and some political savvy to develop strategies to obtain physician input in the most expedient manner possible.

## KEY POINTS IN POLICY DEVELOPMENT

When you actually sit down to write structure standards, consider five key points. These are the nuts and bolts of policy development:

| | |
|---|---|
| **BREVITY** | Unit structure must be concise. An average length of the main body of policies for a nursing unit is ten to fifteen pages. |
| **THOROUGHNESS** | Unit structure must be complete and address all nine components of structure at the unit or division level. |
| **ORGANIZATION** | Structure standards are a set of policies, written in an outline, paragraph, or narrative style. They flow logically from broad structural elements to more detailed content covering predefined components. |
| **APPROVAL/REVIEW** | All structure must show the date and mechanism of approval to give it legitimacy |

CONSISTENCY

and clout. Annual review and authorizing bodies must be evident to meet JCAH requirements and insure continued relevancy.

While you can use policy development to create positive change, you cannot violate or contradict existing policy elsewhere in the system. Familiarize yourself with hospital, administrative, departmental, and medical staff policy to prevent this error.

Dividing Structure standards into general policy and addenda helps to comply with these five points. General policy makes up the main body of your unit policies and provides an overall framework for your Structure standards. Information is broad and seldom changes with time. Addenda are specific policies which provide more detail on topics covered in the general policies.

The word "addendum" means additional, so that an addendum policy is one which is supplemental. Dividing Structure standards into general policy and specific addenda makes the main body of the policies readable in less than an hour. Refer the reader to more specific content in addenda should that information be desired or necessary. The addenda are lettered alphabetically A through Z and are discussed in the related section of the general policy. In the standards manual, which we will discuss later, the general unit policies would appear first, followed by the alphabetically arranged addenda. Examples of addenda topics might be specific unit measures for infection control, exact lists of emergency medications and equipment maintained on a nursing unit, precise staffing and scheduling patterns, the roles of nursing students on your unit, and other matters that often change or require frequent revision. Addenda might also be used to refer the reader to other existing policy for the hospital or department of nursing. An example of general unit structure and reference to an addendum might be: "The 8 West head nurse defines and has responsibility for adhering to the 8 West staff patterns (see addendum F)."

Review general policies annually; rewriting shouldn't be necessary. Your specific addenda, however, may be modified as often as needed to reflect changes or to incorporate new issues that require Structure standards. The point is that setting up your unit structure in these two sections has several advantages. When it's time for revision, it's easier to change one or two pages of addenda than ten pages of general policy. When orienting new staff to your unit policies, it's reasonable for them to review ten to fifteen pages in one sitting and learn what specific addenda exist for later reference than it is to try to absorb 80 plus pages. Finally, staff and managers alike can use the referenced addenda system quickly and expediently to locate information needed for decision making. Table 3-1 lists the characteristics of general policy and addenda.

## CONTENT OF STRUCTURE STANDARDS

Content of policy is limited to the defined elements of structure. Since structure standards need to exist for the department of nursing as an entity and each unit or division as a subsystem of the department, issues to be addressed reflect

## TABLE 3-1
## General Policy versus ADDENDA

| GENERAL POLICIES | ADDENDA |
|---|---|
| • Organized as a set of policies around defined elements of structure (13 at Department of Nursing level; 9 at Nursing Unit level). | • Organized in referenced order as an extension of general policies. |
| • Contains broad policy information. | • Contains specific information. |
| • Written in outline/paragraph style with pages numbered consecutively and alphabetical references to addenda. | • Written in paragraph style on one or more pages, each labeled both by TITLE OF THE ADDENDUM and alphabetical reference (example: "Addendum C: Unit Staffing Patterns"). |
| • Remains fairly constant, with minimal revision year to year. | • Updated as necessary (yearly minimum) to reflect details of new system and respond to frequent or new policy changes. |
| • Kept at a reasonable length (50-60 pages at DON level; 10-15 pages at unit level) | • May be as long as necessary. |
| • Capable of being read and reviewed in a single setting | • Cannot be read in a single setting—serves as reference to managers and staff when requiring detail on a specific policy topic. |

the level of organizational focus. As Chapter Two briefly listed, there are thirteen elements of structure for building policy for the department of nursing and nine elements for the nursing unit or division. These elements are applicable regardless of size or nature of the system. While size may contribute to complexity or simplicity of policy development, the conditions and mechanisms required to run a 1000 bed department of nursing and 60 bed units are the same as needed to manage a 100 bed department and 15 bed units.

Our discussions and examples of content in this book will be limited to unit or division level structure. The better developed the department of nursing Structure standards, the easier will be writing policy for the nursing units. The department structure forms the **Generic** background from which more **Unit Specific** policy can be developed. From here on, department of nursing structure standards will be called "Department of Nursing Generic Policy." The term *generic* means *applicable to all nursing units that make up the department*. The unit division level structure standards will be referred to by that name. Table 3-2 compares the thirteen departmental elements of structure with the nine for a unit.

While the outlines for the elements of structure for the department of nursing and unit appear to have similarities, there is no duplication or conflict. The former is more extensive and broad as it is directed at the operation of an entire department. The latter is more concise and specific because it addresses only the function of a particular sub-system. The unit policies may refer to the generic structure when appropriate to avoid unnecessary repetition. There will be two sets of Structure standards on each nursing area: the generic department of nursing policies in one manual and the specific unit or division policies in another manual. This separation of GENERIC and UNIT SPECIFIC reduces volume, prevents duplication, and increases relevancy. What is written in unit specific policy and available to unit staff is pertinent to that unit only.

Each of the nine elements of structure for the nursing unit or division can be broken down into components for writing policy statements. Subsequent chapters in this unit will address each element, discussing its components and content. Examples will appear for each element. These are generally limited to a Medical-Surgical unit but can easily be altered to apply to Critical Care, Maternal Child Health, or Psychiatry. The reader should know that the content examples in the chapters are abbreviated. A complete set of unit level Structure standards can be found under "Structure" in the Sample Unit Standards Manual at the end of the book.

When addressing each of the nine elements of structure be sure to include statements that address each of the critical components. Table 3-3 lists the components of each element.

## TABLE 3-2

### Elements of Structure

| DEPARTMENT OF NURSING | NURSING UNIT-LEVEL |
|---|---|
| I. Description of Hospital and Department of Nursing. | I. Description of Nursing unit/division. |
| II. Overall Purpose of Department of Nursing. | II. Overall Purpose of unit/division. |
| III. Philosophy of Department of Nursing. | III. Overall Objectives of unit/division. |
| IV. Overall Objectives of Department of Nursing. | IV. Administration/Organization of unit/division. |
| V. Administration/Organization of Department of Nursing. | V. Hours of Operation of unit/division. |
| VI. Hours of Operation of Department of Nursing. | VI. Utilization of the area (admission, duration of stay, transfer, discharge, criteria and planning). |
| VII. Utilization of Patient Care Areas. | VII. Governing Rules of the unit/division. |
| VIII. Utilization of Nursing Staff/Staffing. | VIII. Staffing of the unit/division. |
| IX. Maintenance of a Professional Practice System. | IX. Nursing Responsibilities on the unit/division. |
| X. Governing Rules for Department of Nursing. | |
| XI. Selection/Orientation/Development/Evaluation/Credentialing of Nursing Personnel. | |
| XII. Quality Assurance Activities within Department of Nursing. | |
| XIII. Nursing Responsibilities Across the Department of Nursing. | |

TABLE 3-3

## Structural Elements for
## Unit/Division Standards

I. DESCRIPTION
   A. Location/size
   B. Patient population/acuity
   C. Type of unit

II. PURPOSE

III. OBJECTIVES

IV. ADMINISTRATION/ORGANIZATION
   A. Organizational chart
   B. Narrative
   C. Policy Statements
      1. Nursing direction
      2. Medical direction
      3. Committee structure

V. HOURS OF OPERATION
   A. Regular
   B. Emergency

VI. UTILIZATION OF THE AREA
   A. Admission
      1. Who
      2. How
      3. Circumstances
      4. Criteria
      5. Limitations
      6. Demand for beds beyond capacity
   B. Length of Stay
   C. Transfer/Discharge
      1. When/Who
      2. Planning
      3. Criteria

VII. GOVERNING RULES
   A. General safety
   B. Electrical safety and maintenance
   C. Infection control
   D. Patient valuables
   E. Confidentiality/Patients rights
   F. Supplies/Special equipment
   G. Patient Support services
   H. Fire/Disaster plans

VIII. STAFFING
  A. Quantity
  B. Levels
  C. Delivery of care methodology
  D. Preparation
     1. Selection
     2. Orientation
     3. Continuing education
     4. Credentialing
IX. NURSING RESPONSIBILITIES
  A. RN
  B. LPN
  C. Others

The following chapters adhere to this outline format.

# Chapter 4  Description, Purpose, Objectives, and Administration

The first three elements—the description, purpose, and overall objectives—of your unit can serve as the introduction to your general unit structure. This content defines the broad scope of your unit's services. Here you focus on the fundamental reasons for your unit's existence and your objectives for accomplishment.

## I. DESCRIPTION

The description of your unit addresses location, size, patient population, and type of unit. Simply express these variables in a paragraph. Patient population refers to adults, adolescents, females only, infants, and so forth. Type of unit means the general level of acuity of your patients: critical, acute, convalescent, rehabilitative.

For example:

DESCRIPTION: 8 West is a 40 bed medical/surgical general unit located on the 8th floor of the Main building. It consists of 16 semi-private rooms, and 8 private rooms set up for all types of isolation.

## II. PURPOSE

Under purpose, explain (in one or two sentences) why your unit exists. You may wish to add a statement reflecting your philosophy about nursing care. JCAH requires that departments of nursing have a written philosophy, but does not require that units have one. This section would be the place to state yours. You may say that the unit follows the department of nursing philosophy, without elaboration, or you may choose to state that philosophy, without elaboration, or you may choose to state that philosophy in your own words. You can operationalize your philosophical ideas by writing objectives in the next element.

For example:

PURPOSE: To provide quality care to adult medical/surgical patients who are acutely ill or injured and in varying stages of recuperation from diagnostic, therapeutic, or surgical interventions.

## III. UNIT OBJECTIVES

List the overall objectives your unit strives to achieve. These are unlikely to change from year to year unless the nature of the unit changes, such as in the case of a general medical unit becoming a telemetry stepdown unit. Differentiate these overall unit objectives from your semi-annual management by objectives. Address these four issues in your overall unit objectives: environment, equipment, medical-nursing management, and data collection. After addressing these four areas, you may state any other broad objective related to your unit's specialty or focus, such as research, teaching, or rehabilitation.

For example:

A. To provide an environment conducive to healing through the prompt detection of emergency conditions and through the prevention of complications associated with diseases and disorders; for those patients whose conditions cannot be adequately treated, to provide an environment conducive to death with dignity.

## IV. ADMINISTRATION AND ORGANIZATION

This fourth element of your policies has three parts: the organizational chart for your unit, a descriptive narrative, and the policy statements outlining both the medical and nursing direction of the area and the collaboration of physicians, nurses, and administration through committee structure.

A. Organizational Chart

The organizational chart illustrates the different levels of workers in the unit, and the relationships among them, depicted through lines of communication, accountability, and authority. Solid lines represent a direct supervisory relationship between a particular level and one below it; dotted lines reflect relationships of a collaborative or advisory nature. You may include support personnel, such as clinical specialists and inservice instructors, if they're intimately involved in the unit. Include members of the medical staff who are part of the unit's power base along with the collaborative multi-disciplinary committee.

It's not necessary to include an organizational chart for the entire nursing department, at this will be located in the department of nursing generic standards manual.

B. Narrative

No organizational chart is complete without an accompanying narrative. This is a description of the organizational chart and explains the roles and responsibilities of persons in both supervisory and collaborative positions. Its primary purpose is to prevent incorrect assumptions. Usually, a few sentences are directed at each level of the chart.

Generally, the organizational charts and narrative are not part of the actual policies but are separate sheets of paper placed directly behind the policies. Each has its own labeled tab for quick reference, i.e. "ORGANIZATIONAL CHART (Unit)" and "NARRATIVE". These two pieces separate the set of policies from the alphabetized addenda.

C. Policy Statements

In this section of your structure standards you are creating policy statements that serve as the basis for the organizational chart and narrative just discussed. These statements will be directed toward three issues: the nursing direction of the unit, the medical direction of the unit, and the collaborative process of a multi-disciplinary committee.

*Nursing direction* outlines the levels of supervison for unit operation, staff function, and patient care. This section gives the various levels of nursing management the power they need to do their jobs. It addresses such issues as 24-hour accountability, decentralization, limitations of decision making, overlapping responsibilities between management levels, and contributions of alternate shift supervisory personnel. This content validates information in the organizational chart and narrative by specifically delineating nursing management functions. Content will be directed at four levels of nursing management:

- first line managers and their alternatives;
- middle management;
- executive management; and
- supervisory support staff

For example:

1. Nursing Direction
   a. The 8 West PCS is an RN with appropriate clinical and managerial experience and/or the potential for same. S/he is specially selected by the Nursing Administration to assume responsibility for the effective organization and management of the 8 West area. S/he has 24 hour responsibility for the effective functioning of the staff including development and evaulation; the efficient functioning of the 8 West subsystem; and the quality of patient care provided in the setting.

*Medical direction* is a potentially sensitive but critical area for definition. Here you define responsibilities of the medical staff as they relate to the nursing staff and the nursing unit. This content should be negotiated with the physicians in terms of issues addressed and language used. Variables such as timing, nurse/doctor relationships, and political environment, influence your success here. However, these issues must be clarified through well written policy because each topic frequently frustrates the nursing staff and potentially jeopardizes patient care. The purpose of this content must be clear to both nurses and physicians: it is not aimed at telling physicians how to practice medicine but rather at defining doctor's professional obligations to the nursing staff who provide care to the patients they admit. Four issues (optional fifth) should be addressed here:

- overall physician direction of patient's medical care;
- responsibilities of attending physicians;
- responsibilities of the Medical Director or Service Chiefs;
- responsibilities of physician consultants; and,
- responsibilities of teaching staff (if applicable to your setting).

For example:
   2. Medical Direction
      a. The responsibility for directing medical care on 8 West is that of the Attending (Admitting) Physician and associates. This responsibility may be delegated, but it must be done as specified in the Medical Staff Bylaws, through a written order for transfer of services or by consultation.

Formulate this policy by sitting down with key members of the medical staff and discussing past and current problem situations. Try not to be rigid or threatening and avoid over generalization and nit-picking! Deal with facts and keep the focus on the wellbeing of the nursing staff and patients. Be willing to negotiate and compromise on phraseology but get these issues defined to minimize unit and nurse abuse. What's "nurse abuse"? Things like physicians' admitting patients to a unit and not seeing them until several hours or a day later; or writing illegible orders and progress notes which contribute to confusion or error by the nursing staff; or expecting nurses to set up initial physician to physician consultation; or expecting nursing staff to "resolve" conflicts among and between consulting physicians; or wasting valuable nursing hours through unneccessary phone calls for clarification of medical direction or extensive "updates" to physicians "taking call" for other physicians. Read through the issues above very carefully, and you will see that they address simply professional courtesy and minimal legal definition of safe medical practice in communication with and direction of nurses.

### Attending Physicians

Begin by stating who has primary responsibility for patients admitted to your unit. In some hospitals, the attending physician may not be the same doctor whose name appears on the admission sheet because of the duties of the teaching staff. Then describe key responsibilities of the primary physician in relation to the admitting unit and nursing staff. Address the following areas:

- seeing patients on admission and on what basis afterwards;
- directing the nursing staff in carrying out medical care plans;
- writing clear, legible orders;
- completing the required medical documentation (H&P, progress records);
- collaborating with the nursing staff, the patient, and the patient's family;
- being available to the nursing staff when needed;
- signing out to other physicians;
- participating in staff development, care conferences, and standards development;
- preventing or clarifying conflicts with consultants.

### Medical Director/Chief of Service

Medical directors are usually found directing critical care units. Reiterate the directors responsibilities as they're spelled out in the JCAH standards for special care, but express them in your own words, with focus on your unit. Your content will revolve around four key Director responsibilities: (1) bed utilization, (2) implementation of special care unit and medical staff policy, (3) quality assurance activities, and (4) medical and nursing staff continuing education. For units outside the critical care areas where the position of a medical director probably doesn't exist, aim the policies at the chief of the service, such as the Chief of Medicine, Surgery, or Obstetrics. The medical staff bylaws usually address the roles of the chiefs of service.

Generally, the role of a service chief is troubleshooting, working with medical quality assurance, and coordinating continuing education for doctors on their service. With respect to their relationship with nurses, however, service chiefs are not required to police the doctors under them. Traditionally, this has been the unwritten, unspoken job of nursing—one that nursing isn't paid to do and one that causes endless trouble.

Most managers have their hands full dealing with strictly nursing problems. That's why you must work with your directors of nursing to define the role of service chiefs in relation to nursing. Their responsibilities (as well as those of the medical director in a critical care unit) should include:

- being available to nursing managers for problem-solving when controversial issues of medical management arise on nursing units (and the patient's personal physician is not available);
- dealing with doctors when direct confrontation by the nursing manager has failed to produce results;
- helping to create and maintain nurse-physician liaison committees;
- assisting with the development of standards and their approval so that they have the support of the medical staff.

Not to tap the power, assistance, and support in the person of your service chief is foolish. You would only continue to experience frustration and burnout from being placed in the impossible position of trying to do something that no nurse can do—hold physicians accountable for their own responsibilities.

## Physician Consultants

Now turn your attention to defining the responsibilities of physician consultants. Again, the key issues to address are:

- clear and complete documentation including orders and progress notes;
- availability to the nursing staff;
- collaboration with the patient and family;
- collaboration with the attending physician to prevent conflicting direction to the nursing staff.

Clarification of this content can prevent nurses from being caught up in "physician activities."

## Teaching Staff

If you work in a teaching hospital—with interns, residents, and other house staff—you must clarify several potentially problematic issues common to your setting. Often nurses must contend with shifts in medical direction and new regimens of therapy whenever the teaching staff rotates. To avoid confusion during the integration of new physicians into your system, your Structure standards should specifically discuss:

- the hierarchy of the teaching staff;
- special conduct regulations (such as name tages, dress code);
- publication of coverage;
- availability of house staff to nursing units;
- appropriate direction of the nursing staff and participation in nursing continuing education;
- collaboration with medical staff to prevent conflicts;
- interaction with the patient and family;
- mutual responsibilities (such as IV's, drug administration, blood administration, emergency measures);
- adherance to unit standards.

This section of your general policies should be shared with the medical staff office as a basis for orienting new doctors, whether they're permanent members of the medical staff or temporary teaching staff members.

Examples of these standards can be found in the Sample Unit Standards Manual.

*Committee Structure* discusses the formation of a liaison committee, perhaps one of the most important aspects of this section of your unit policies. Each nursing division should form such a committee, so that selected members of the nursing management team, medical staff, and administration can meet regularly to discuss the operation of the unit and patient care. The word "liaison" implies a close working relationship for the purpose of collaboration and communication. The committee provides a forum for negotiating controversial patient care issues, serves as a basis for improving communication, and fosters relationships characterized by trust, respect, and mutual understanding. Eventually, the committee may evolve into a multi-disciplinary quality assurance group.

In creating policy for such a committee, address the following:

- name and nature of the committee (ad hoc or standing);
- its purpose;
- members (official and *ex officio*);
- chairperson (or co-chairpersons);
- method of selecting members and chairperson;
- preparation of agendas;
- documentation of minutes.

The liaison committee should be a permanent group of selected members of the nursing, medical, and administrative staff who meet monthly (or at least quarterly) to collaborate on difficult care issues, to develop and approve standards, and to discuss quality assurance activities. Members of the committee should include key representatives of the medical staff, such as chiefs of service and other doctors who use the units extensively and have a vested interest in seeing them operate efficiently. Nursing committee members should be first-line managers, their assistants or charge nurses, clinical specialists or instructors, the middle manager of the division, and possibly department heads who have a close working relationship with the units.

To save time and avoid duplication of effort, it's usually best to form liaison committees at the division level, such as a Medical-Surgical Liaison Committee, Maternal-Child Health Liaison Committee, Mental-Psych Health Committee, and so forth. Such committees facilitate coordination among units dealing with similar patient populations and staff. Assigning a nurse and a physician as co-chairpersons will serve to equalize power and ensure that both the nursing and medical staffs are fairly represented.

Finally, you can consider other committees and meetings that are used to operate your area. For instance, you might briefly discuss the unit's contributions to Department of Nursing Committees such as the Standards Committee, or Quality Assurance Committee. You might also include internal unit meetings such as staff meeting and care conferences.

# Chapter 5 Hours of Operation and Utilization

## V. HOURS OF OPERATION

This brief element in your unit structure can be completed by specifying when your area is "open for business", so to speak. Some units are open 24 hours a day, but those that are not must have Policies that clearly spell out their hours of operation and special considerations for staffing coverage. Nursing units can be divided into bedded and non-bedded units. A bedded unit is staffed to deliver around-the-clock care and thus is open 24 hours a day. Two factors—the number of hours of nursing care (HNC) provided by the unit and its average daily census (ADC)—are used to determine the number of nurses needed to staff the unit properly. Of course, allowances must also be made for the acuity level of the patients on the unit. But basically, if you use HNC and ADC to staff, your unit is a bedded unit, and all you need to define your hours of operation is a statement doing so.

For example:

8 West is a bedded unit providing set hours of care to an average daily census 24 hours a day. Staffing will be adjusted for census changes and increased or decreased acuity levels among the patients on the unit.

Non-bedded units, however, don't have an average daily census or a set number of hours of nursing care. They function according to varying patient loads or by the clock. Since these units may not be open 24 hours a day, their policies must state specific hours of operation, including regular and emergency hours; alternate mechanisms to provide similar care during "off" hours; and staffing measures. Examples of such units are the emergency room, operating room, recovery room, labor and delivery areas, and ambulatory or outpatient service areas. When are these units open for patient care? When are these units closed? Is there an "on call" system? How does it work? What are the requirements and limitations of personnel who are on call? Although some of these units are open 24 hours a day, they're not staffed for maximum volume—for example, the emergency room, or the labor and delivery area. The need for extra staffing to help handle an unusually high number of patients can be briefly mentioned in this subsection, with more specific details reserved for the staffing section of your Structure standards.

For example:

POST ANESTHESIA RECOVERY ROOM

I. Hours of Operation
   A. Regular hours of operation for this unit are 8:00 A.M. to 8:30 P.M., Monday through Friday. On Saturday, the unit is open from 8:00 A.M. to 4:30 P.M.
   B. Emergency hours are between 8:30 P.M. and 8:00 A.M., Monday through Friday, between 4:30 P.M. and 8:00 A.M. on Saturdays, and all Sundays and holidays. The unit will be covered during these hours by the PAR staff as specified in:
      1. "Policy for Delivery of Care" (see addendum A);
      2. "On-Call Policy" (see addendum B);
      3. "Policy for Immediate Postoperative Recovery of Patients" (see addendum C).

Note how this example demonstrates the proper use of addenda to distinguish between general unit Policies and specific addenda. Addenda A, B, and C provide more detailed information on how the unit functions during emergency periods.

VI. UTILIZATION OF THE UNIT

This element of your policies is extensive and important because it specifies how your unit will be used by nurses, doctors, patients, and the admitting office. It consists of three subsections:

A. Admission policies,
B. Length of stay policies,
C. Transfer/discharge policies.

Unless your policies state how your unit is to be used, the unit stands a very good chance of being abused. If utilization of your unit has never been defined, utilization can be open to anyone's interpretation and you may find yourself trying to be all things to all people—patients, doctors, other nurses, and other departments.

# ADMISSION POLICIES

In this first subsection, you should address six key questions regarding the manner in which patients are admitted to your unit:

1.) Which doctors can admit patients?
2.) How are patients admitted?
3.) What information should be contained in medical orders on admission?
4.) What are the criteria for admission?
5.) What are the limitations of your unit?
6.) How does your unit deal with a demand for beds beyond its capacity?

If you answer these questions adequately, you will have clearly specified the proper manner in which your unit is to be used.

***Which doctors can admit patients to your unit?*** A statement pointing out which doctors have admission privileges on your unit; the difference between regular and courtesy privileges; and the requirements for consultation will answer this first question. Since this information concerns medical rules and regulations, it should be clearly spelled out in the medical staff bylaws. Use them as a reference for writing this policy to help nurses when admitting patients at odd hours or when dealing with a new doctor.

For example:

All members of the medical staff with active admitting privileges may admit patients to 8 West. Doctors with courtesy privileges must be approved by the Chief of Service

***How are patients admitted to your unit?*** This question can be answered by using the D-E-T-R (Direct, Emergency, Transfer, Routine) approach to categorize admissions to bedded units:

Direct-    Specify just who these patients are and how they get to your unit. Do they come from the emergency room or admissions office? Are they strictly ambulance admissions? Are there some acutely ill patients who should not be direct admissions because it would be too dangerous?

For example:

Direct Admissions
    are admitted directly from their doctor's offices or their homes with arrangements made by phone through the admissions office. These patients may transport themselves to the hospital, or they may arrive on the unit with medical orders. These orders may be written by the patient's doctor and brought to the unit by the patient himself, or they may be written in the emergency room after an initial medical assessment there. Medical orders relayed by

telephone before the patient's arrival on the unit will also be acceptable for admission.

Emergency-Briefly discuss the acuity level of patients transferred to your unit from the emergency room. Also note any special requirements for these patients, such as being accompanied by a qualified escort or requiring specified equipment.

For example:

Emergency Admissions
are patients admitted from the emergency room. These patients must also arrive on the unit with medical orders, written by the emergency room physician or relayed by telephone to the unit by the Attending Physician.

Transfer- Generally, transfer patients are postoperative and post-code patients; in addition, transfers often take place between critical care and noncritical care units. Address the mechanisms by which these admissions take place.

For example:

Transfer patients
are admitted to 8 West from other units, such as the intensive care unit, the coronary care unit, or the operating room. The unit transferring the patient must obtain updated medical orders before the transfer and insure that these orders accompany the patient to the unit.

Routine- Because these patients are elective admissions, scheduled in advance, their acuity level should be low. Thus their entry into your unit may be handled by the admitting office, a volunteer, or even family members. Outline these mechanisms of admission.

For example:

Routine admissions
are patients scheduled in advance for admission to 8 West. These patients may be brought to the unit by admitting clerks or volunteer workers with written medical orders. The Admitting Officer must obtain these orders or alert the nursing staff on the unit if orders have not been written so that the Attending Physician can be contacted. Physicians are strongly encouraged to send routine admissions to the nursing unit with prewritten medical orders.

Two other categories of admission that need to be discussed in this section are **boarders** and **overflow** patients. Boarders are patients who don't belong on your unit, but who occupy one of your beds because no bed is available on the appropriate unit. These patients should be flagged on admission and moved as soon as a bed on the appropriate unit is available. Requesting nursing consultations and sharing relevant nursing standards with the appropriate unit will help you manage the care of these patients until they can be transferred.

Overflow patients fall into the opposite category. They belong on your unit but because no beds are available, they have to be admitted to another unit. In such cases, your policies should allow you to request that the most stable patient on your unit be transferred in exchange for the overflow patient who has a greater need for your services.

Although policies relating to boarders and overflow patients aren't meant to be rigidly interpreted, they do make a strong statement about nursing care in your institution by making it clear that patients have special needs that can best be met on designated nursing units. These policies reinforce the importance of admitting patients to the institution on units where the nursing staff can best manage and provide the care they need.

Examples of policies regarding boarders and overflow patients are outlined in the Sample Unit Standards Manual.

Non-bedded areas can categorize their admissions in a similar manner but will have to "brainstorm" the methods of entry into their respective areas. For example in the OR, categories of admission would be related to the various functions of the operating room and the posting mechanisms and should address the following areas: holding areas and anesthesia induction areas; routine elective cases; emergency cases; local or diagnostic cases.

For the Post Anesthesia Recovery Room, categories would be directed at the use of the PAR and entry mechanisms. They would address: preoperative holding areas for teaching, sedation, or invasive line insertion; special areas set aside for pediatric, post anesthesia delirium patients, or infected patients; general post surgical-anesthesia patients; local anesthesia patients.

The Emergency Room would address the various mechanisms of entry such as: the triage patients as urgent, emergent, and non-emergent and their immediate care or referral; walk-ins; registered or unregistered obstetric patients; direct admissions; ambulance admissions.

Finally, an outpatient area could designate its utilization by addressing its various functions: out patient day surgery; local procedures done in the area; private physicians visits; follow-up non-emergency clinic appointment activities; and gastro-enterology procedures.

***What information should be contained in medical orders on admission?***
Here you should list precisely what type of medical orders you need before patitents can be admitted to your unit. This is a critical issue for all nursing units and must be clearly defined for protection of patients. No patient should be on your unit for any length of time without adequate medical direction. Such an oversight can jeopardize staff efficiency and patient care. At least eight areas must be included in admission medical orders:

1. Admitting diagnosis and order to admit to unit;
2. Code status and directions for the management of a life-threatening crisis;
3. Diet;

4. Activity level;
5. Vital signs (and how often they should be taken);
6. Laboratory tests that need to be scheduled;
7. Routine medication (especially those the patient takes on his own);
8. PRN medications (analgesics, laxatives, antacids, and so forth).

You may want to include your prerequisites on standardized, preprinted physician admission order forms. You could then have the sheets distributed to the doctor's offices, the emergency room, and any other area from which patients may be admitted. This arrangement will make it easier for doctors to provide you with the information you need and will help ensure comprehensive admission orders for all patients.

In this subsection, you must also specify when the doctor is to see newly admitted patients. Other pertinent topics for discussion would be the need for physician documentation on admission including an admission note, a patient history, and physical examination findings, and nursing responsibilities on admitting, including collaboration with the admission office about where the patient should be placed on the unit, and entry of the patient's name into the unit log book.

*What are the criteria for admission?* To answer this fourth question, you need to define your patient population by specifying the types of patients for whom you provide care on your unit. Admission criteria may be described by the patient's physical state, the level of care he requires, or his medical diagnosis. General descriptions like "acutely ill adult medical-surgical patients" imply that patients who are critically ill, or who are below a certain age, or who belong on a special unit, are not candidates for admission to your unit. But the more specific you can be the better. If you or your chief of service prefers to avoid specific medical diagnoses, you can write general criteria for admission such as:

- dependency on essential or life-support equipment (such as artificial airways or ventilators, peritoneal dialysis, intravenous lines or any other essential equipment common to your area);
- unstable hemodynamic measurements or vital signs requiring continuous monitoring and frequent nursing interventions (for example, strict monitoring of fluid and electrolyte status, frequent vital signs, or intravenous pain management);
- acute illness or traumatic injury requiring diagnostic or therapeutic medical and nursing intervention (here you could list common examples from among your patient population);
- abnormal laboratory values (such as abnormal ABG's, unstable blood glucose, BUN, or electrolyte levels, or elevated cardiac or liver enzymes) contributing to unstable body systems.

For example:

4. Criteria for admission
   a. Generally, a patient is considered a candidate for admission to 8 West if he is an adult experiencing an acute or potentially acute

illness or injury, or an exacerbation of a chronic condition, affecting one or more body system.
  b. Common candidates for admission include:
    1) Post-ICU transfer patients from both medical and surgical units;
    2) Patients with diseases or disorders requiring diagnostic or therapeutic intervention, such as diabetes mellitus, gastrointestinal bleeding, abdominal pain, chronic obstructive pulmonary disease, and congestive heart failure;
    3) Post-op general anesthesia and local surgical and orthopaedic patients;
    4) Patients transferred from cardiac stepdown units;
    5) Patients receiving total parenteral nutrition;
    6) Patients with chronic renal failure who may need hemodialysis.

*What are the limitations of your unit?* Asking yourself this question will prompt you to define the types of patients or situations that your unit is not prepared to handle. Every unit has its own limitations as far as:
  • physical environment or available equipment,
  • acuity level of patients,
  • the skills of its nursing staff.

Stating the limitations of your unit will prevent your staff from being placed in situations that they're not qualified to handle—and not expected to handle. It will also reduce the risk of patients' receiving inferior nursing care because they've been placed on the wrong unit.

For example:

5. Limitations
  a. 8 West has only 8 private rooms for the isolation of patients with infectious diseases or reduced resistance to disease.

*How does your unit deal with a demand for beds beyond its capacity?* Occasionally, the situation will arise in which your unit has no empty beds but there are still patients who could benefit from being placed there. It's a good idea to spell out the steps for the staff and nursing managers to follow under such circumstances. On critical care units it's more than a good idea—it's a JCAH requirement, but all nursing units can benefit. Key issues, such as collaboration with the admissions office, the nursing management team, and chief of service can be covered. If doctors should be called to make beds available, consider the most expeditious use of nurses' time. Spending too much time on the phone trying to shuffle beds can be avoided by defining how your resources are to be used and delineating the responsibilities of key personnel such as nursing office supervisors and the admitting officer on duty.

For example:

6. Demand for Beds Beyond Capacity
  a. The capacity of 8 West is 40 beds. When the patient census ex-

ceeds the budgeted daily census, the shift coordinator will notify the Patient Care Supervisor (PCS) or Nursing Office Supervisor (NOS).

b. The shift coordinator will consult the admissions office early each day to validate potential or scheduled discharges and anticipated admissions. She will also collaborate with the admission office on determining the number, time of admission, and placement of patients.

c. If the admissions office or the emergency room need to place a patient on 8 West and no bed is available, the shift coordinator and admitting officer will collaborate with the chief of service to transfer or discharge an appropriate 8 West patient. The NOS will address staffing needs accordingly.

## LENGTH OF STAY POLICIES

This relatively brief subsection should follow your admission policies. Its purpose is to identify how the length of a patient's stay on your unit is monitored and controlled through daily collaboration between the nursing and medical staffs, an important issue with the advent of DRG's. Here you can point out what your unit is doing to shorten lengths of stay and to deal with extended lengths of stay beyond what your institution has determined to be acceptable. Spell out specific measures, such as the need for medical documentation of complications in cases involving extended lengths of stay, the Utilization Review Committee's role on your unit, and the use of discharge planning rounds or services that can facilitate the discharge process.

For example:

B. Length of Stay Policies
   1. Generally, length of stay is determined by the patient's physical status and his ability to perform self care, as determined by the Attending Physician and the nursing staff.

## DISCHARGE/TRANSFER POLICIES

This third and final subsection of Structure standards outlining the use of your unit will discuss transfer and discharge policies. Here you need to address such issues as:

- the need for discharge orders;
- criteria for discharge or transfer and documented evidence that the patient has met them;
- daily assessment of a patient's readiness for discharge by the nursing and medical staffs, and documentation of this collaboration;
- multidisciplinary discharge planning rounds (conference);
- mechanisms for discharging or transferring patients to another nursing unit;

- maintenance of the unit log book, to track disposition, length of stay, and complications.

Perhaps the most important of these issues is the criteria for discharge. By definition, a patient is ready for discharge when he no longer meets your admission criteria. If you've already defined your admission criteria clearly in the earlier subsection of policies, you should be able to easily reverse them to formulate your discharge criteria. Discharge criteria can be established on a broad level so they will apply to all of your patients and then be individualized from patient to patient by nursing staff and physicians. Usually criteria for transfer from an area of the hospital revolve around six issues. Patients are considered candidates for transfer/discharge when nurse-physician collaboration determines that patients demonstrate:

- no need for essential or life support equipment,
- no need for therapeutic measures provided by nursing staff,
- stable vital body systems and no need for frequent or continuous monitoring,
- stable significant lab values,
- satisfactory psychological coping abilities,
- satisfactory cognitive abilities for self care.

For example:

7. Discharge Criteria from 8 West are:
   a. The patient achieves independence from life support equipment such as peritoneal dialysis, IV therapy, indwelling lines (unless to be sent home with supportive care).
   b. The patient achieves independence from therapeutic measures performed by nursing or support services (unless these are to be continued at home with assistance).

These discharge/transfer criteria can be printed onto a nursing form and incorporated into the patients' record where they can be consulted daily. As nurse-physician interaction evaluates that the patient has met a criterion, it is checked off. Such a record provides an objective yardstick for determining when a patient is really ready to leave a unit or go home. It validates multidisplinary efforts to prepare patients for discharge and gives evidence that the patients are indeed ready for discharge. This approach maximizes effective use of beds by discouraging excessive stay lengths while simultaneously preventing premature discharge. This type of record also indicates when a patient is discharged without meeting a discharge criterion and documents that follow-up referral has been provided.

# Chapter 6 Governing Rules of the Unit

## VII. GOVERNING RULES

This element of your structure standards concerns physical, environmental, and safety issues, always key factors in JCAH accreditation. Each topic discussed here is appears in the JCAH hospital accreditation manual in its nursing service standards. Eight topics should be addressed:

- General safety,
- Electrical safety and maintenance,
- Infection control,
- Patient valuables,
- Confidentiality, and patient rights,
- Emergency equipment and supplies,
- Patient support services,
- Fire and disaster plans.

The actual content in this section needn't be lengthy, since some of these topics are addressed elsewhere—in hospital, department of nursing, and infection control policies. By taking the time to spell out your unit's policy with regard to these governing rules, however, you can reinforce compliance with these overall policies. At the same time you can focus on specific measures devised by your unit to augment the content that already exists. You can thus tailor the policies to fit your unit, patient population, and staff. Much content in this section will be in unit specific addenda.

Let's take a look at each of the topics to be covered in this section.

## A. GENERAL SAFETY

Address precisely what you and your staff do about regulating the number of visitors and hospital employees on your unit. If you follow the department of nursing policy or the hospital policy on visiting hours to the letter, then say so in this subsection. Allow for occasional modification of existing policies to provide exceptions, for example, to restrict enforcement of visiting hours for family members. Define measures to control the traffic on your unit. Remember that such units as the operating room and the labor and delivery area are not the only places that must consider the increased risk of infection created by congestion at the nursing stations and in the hallways. Now is also a good time to address smoking restrictions on your unit and any limitations on private-duty nurses. Review the safety measures you've taken to ensure that all patients are properly identified and to prevent medication errors and patient/employee accidents. Discuss the use of incident reports, special safety concerns in patient transport, noise control, and limitations on "clutter" in the patient care areas. In general, the more you can spell out safety issues, the more effective your unit risk management will be. You can address these matters generally in several brief paragraphs and supplement them with details in an addendum on "Safety Policies."

For example:

A. General Safety
1. Visitor traffic control:
   a. Visiting hours and regulations on 8 West are those specified in department of nursing and hospital policies.
   b. The nursing staff on the unit may alter these visiting hours and regulations based on the patient's condition. Security personnel are available to help control unruly or problem visitors.

## B. ELECTRICAL SAFETY AND MAINTENANCE

Under this subsection, describe your special precautions for electrically sensitive patients. "Electrically sensitive" refers to any patient who because of his condition or therapy is vulnerable to stray electrical currents and thus at risk of being electrocuted. Examples would be patients with pacemakers or pulmonary artery lines or any patient connected to multiple pieces of electrical equipment simultaneously. Also define measures used to protect staff from electrical hazards and educational updates to keep them informed of such measures. Next, briefly outline the routine maintenance activities for keeping essential equipment in working order. Note who keeps maintenance records and where they are stored for reference.

For example:

B. Electrical Safety and Maintenance:
1. The Biomedical Department will perform regularly scheduled maintenance on portable defibrillators and monitors, electrical

beds, diagnostic equipment, EKG machines, and other electrical equipment. Maintenance records will be kept by the PCS as part of 8 West Quality Assurance Activities and in the Biomedical Department.
2. Electrical safety standards for 8 West are summarized in Addendum B.

## C. INFECTION CONTROL

Even though all nursing departments have infection control policies, each unit should briefly outline its specific measures to prevent infection and cross contamination. The best way handle this is to refer to department policy with general statements and use addenda to outline more detailed infection control measures for your patient population and staff. Brainstorm what factors place your patients at high risk for infection and cross contamination. Then define measures used to minimize these factors.

For example:

C. Infection Control:
  1. 8 West adheres to appropriate infection control measures outlined in Department of Nursing Infection Control Manual.
  2. Patients requiring isolation procedures may be admitted to 8 West if proper isolation measures ie. private room can be accommodated as necessary.
  3. Specific Infection Control Measures for 8 West may be found in Addendum C.

## D. PATIENT VALUABLES

In this subsection, specify how your unit handles patient valuables. If this content is adequately addressed in generic department of Nursing Policies, refer the reader to them and summarize the content briefly. But if your nursing unit is one where the risk of losing a patient's valuables is high—the emergency room or the labor and delivery area, for example—you'll want to add more detail and identify specific control measures. Also, emphasize the safekeeping of commonly misplaced patient articles (such as eyeglasses, dentures, and prostheses) that lead to patient complaints and financial loss for the hospital.

For example:

D. Patient Valuables:
  1. Patients valuables are handled according to departmental and hospital policy.
  2. Patients are discouraged from keeping jewelry or more than five dollars in cash in their rooms.

## E. CONFIDENTIALITY AND PATIENT RIGHTS

The topics of patient confidentiality and bill of rights are usually covered in generic departmental or hospital policy, so appropriate reference to existing policy would be all that's needed here. You may include existing policy as an addendum or simply state where the policy can be found. Because confidentiality is a serious ethical issue, go on to emphasize certain matters, such as inquiries from new media, patients' seeing their own records, nurses acting as witnesses, access to patient records, warnings about casual staff communication in public areas, and so forth.

For example:

E. Patient Confidentiality and Patients Rights:
1. All patient information is considered confidential and is protected by the hospital's Patient Bill of Rights.
2. Any discussion of patient information in public areas is a violation of hospital policy, requiring disciplinary action.

## F. EMERGENCY EQUIPMENT AND SUPPLIES

In this subsection you want to address some important questions:

- What emergency equipment (such as a crash cart, cardiac monitor, EKG machine, and defibrillator) is kept on your unit? Where is it kept?
- How is this equipment maintained? How and where is maintenance documented? How is the equipment replaced?
- Where are the emergency drugs kept? Stock drugs and routine supplies? Who provides backup?

You may supplement your answers to these questions with checklists and a unit diagram showing the location of emergency equipment and supplies and safety devices, such as fire extinguishers. Don't forget to specify how your crash cart is checked. Including your crash cart checklist as an addendum is a good idea; besides listing what is available in emergencies, it'll show that you check the cart regularly. (JCAH special care unit standard require that crash carts be check during each nursing shift and the emergency equipment in all other units be checked every 24 hours.)

For example:

F. Emergency Equipment and Supplies:
1. Emergency equipment and supplies on 8 West include a crash cart, emergency drugs, and intubation equipment. Emergency trays can be found on the crash cart. (See Addendum D for crash cart checklist).

## G. PATIENT SUPPORT SERVICES

In this very brief subsection, simply state the emergency and routine laboratory, diagnostic, and blood bank services available to your unit. Also, describe the method by which hemodialysis is available for patients who need it. This content verifies that as an acute care area, your nursing unit has timely access to those patient support services. Thus, you can take appropriate actions if these services fail to meet the needs of the patients, physicians, or nursing staff. (You may have an addendum to this section if you wish.)

For example:

G. Patient Support Services:
    1. 8 West has ready access to emergency and routine laboratory, diagnostic radiology, and blood bank services on a 24 hour basis. In accordance with department of nursing policy, the term *stat* will be reserved for life threatening or potential patient deterioration states as defined by the medical staff.

## H. FIRE AND DISASTER PLANS

Finally, the governing rules of your unit must address the role it plays in hospital fire and disaster plans. Briefly mention how the staff is oriented and reviewed on these plans, since both topics are mandated by JCAH for staff development. Include mention of evacuation routes and direction of such measure by an overall disaster coordinator.

For example:

H. Fire and Disaster Plans:
    1. All staff will participate in unit orientation related to the role of nursing personnel and 8 West in hospital fire and disaster plans.

# Chapter 7  Staffing and Nursing Responsibilities

These last two elements will complete your unit structure standards. The staffing content in particular is complex and likely to require several addenda to present the extensive information needed.

## VIII. STAFFING

In order to ensure a comprehensive discussion of this structural element, you must address four aspects:

- Quantity,
- Levels,
- Delivery of Care Methodology,
- Preparation.

### A. QUANTITY

*Quantity* refers to the number of nurses giving patient care on the unit. Avoid exact numbers in the main body of your policies; instead, state the determining factors for calculating how many nurses you need to deliver effective patient care. Most units are staffed according to full-time equivalents (FTE's), derived from the average daily census of the unit and the hours of nursing care required for each paitent. Historically, hours of nursing care have been based on national averages of patient acuity levels adjusted by the institution's nursing administration. This generally comes to 5 to 8 hours of nursing care per patient in medical/surgical units, and 12 to 16 (or as much as 20 to 24) hours per patient in critical care units. Patient classification systems attempt to refine these figures to arrive at some average acuity level for a unit's patient population. Ideally, they provide a way to determine daily prospective staffing needs, while justifying FTE projections. If your patient acuity changes, it will affect your staffing needs. Also, of course when your census fluctuates above or below ADC, your staffing needs will fluctuate accordingly. So you want to explain the rationale for determining your staffing needs in your general policies, reserving precise numbers and other details for addenda.

This subsection should also address:

- Scheduling practices: How is a time schedule made out for your unit? How is it modified? Who prepares it and in what time frame? How are staff made aware of it? What principles of staffing govern your scheduling practices? Address such mattter as the use of a request book, the maximum number of days that can be worked in a row, the levels of staff that can switch shifts, the use of straight shift system as opposed to a rotation system, and so forth. You may also refer here to generic department of nursing policies.
- Staffing adjustments: When either extreme, too much staff or not enough staff occurs, what adjustments can you make? You want to ensure that nursing managers make fair and consistent decisions on staffing matters, so spell out where and how extra hours of nursing care are provided when your patient census or acuity levels increase, whether through overtime, more part-time personnel, a float/per diem staff, or agency nurses. Also, identify what options the nursing manager or the staff members have regarding too many nurses on duty, days off with or without pay, reassignment to another unit, or assignment to a special project or activity.

For example:

VIII. STAFFING
  A. Quantity
     1. 8 West is staffed with defined number of professional and non-professional staff members to provide the required hours of nursing care for its average daily census as outlined in the annual nursing budget.


  B. LEVELS OF STAFFING

This subsection stipulates who provides care on the unit according to their titles. It reemphasizes the role of the professional nurse in planning, supervising, and evaluating patient care, as required by JCAH nursing service standards. You'll deal here with the limitations of those personnel who are not regular staff members, such as private-duty and student nurses, "float staff," and agency nurses. Specify "Regular staff to non-regular staff" ratio that you feel is safe, spelling out limitations of non-regular staff—restricted patient assignment, for example, or ineligibility for the position of charge nurse. "Floating" policies should be clearly stated since they're controversial and often cause labor-management problems.

Finally, you want to discuss the difference in functions between RN's and LPN's in your unit's delivery mechanism.

For example:

B. Levels
   1. Patient care on 8 West is given by the following levels of staff:
      • RN's,
      • LPN's,
      • NA's,
      • private-duty nurses (RN's or LPN's),
      • clinical specialists,
      • clinical instructors,
      • RN nursing students assisted by their faculty.
   2. Staffing will always provide for no less than 75% of regular unit staff at all times. Non-regular staff members will be assigned only to patients for which they are qualified to care. They will not be made shift coordinators and will at all times work under the direction of the regular staff. They will receive an orientation to the unit and full report by the shift coordinator prior to giving patient care.

## C. DELIVERY OF CARE METHODOLOGY

This subsection of your staffing policies defines how the unit delivers patient care, including the methods used to facilitate communication, coordination, and continuity among staff members and between shifts. These issues must be clear if your unit is to work as a whole, and not as two or three different shifts pulling against each other, undermining the quality of care and creating poor working relationships. The nursing manager can translate ideas into solid plans by giving her staff direction. Answer such questions as:

- What words should be used to describe the unit's delivery of care method? How does this important definition relate to the department of nursing's philosophy care delivery? Can it be unequivocally labeled team, functional, or primary? If not, what is it called? Is your delivery of care method consistent on all shifts?
- How does the method work? Who delivers care using this approach? Both RN's and non-RN's? Just RN's? How is nursing process operationalized using the method?
- When and how are assignments made? By whom? How can assignments be modified? How are unit functional assignments made—for example, narcotics checks or crash cart checks? How are new admissions assigned? Is there co-assignment for non-RN's?
- What is included in shift report? Who attends? How long does it last? Is it taped? Are there indications for "walking rounds" on certain patients? What content should be included and excluded?
- Who is in charge of the unit during each shift? How is this person assigned or appointed? What are his/her responsibilities? Does

he/she take a patient care assignment? Under what circumstances and what acuity? What is the relationship between the charge person and the staff? Between the charge person and the nursing supervisor?

- What are the responsibilities of nonprofessional staff members for communicating, reporting, and documenting? Do they chart on the patient's records or call doctors? Do they sign nurses' notes? Do they contribute information on the Kardex? To what degree are they supervised? How are they held accountable by the professional staff?

These questions deal with critical issues which, if not consistently handled throughout the unit, can disrupt workloads, the supervision of personnel, communications, and working relationships. This subsection can also prove invaluable in orienting new staff members, evaluating staff and charge personnel, and holding staff members accountable for defined responsibilities.

As with previous sections in your structure standards, the issues can be addressed in general terms in the body of your policies and detailed in addenda. If your delivery of care involves any aspect of the team or modular method, you might use a unit diagram to show how the unit breaks down. Of course, any team approach should be related to the Kardex system, patient assignments, and reporting routines.

For example:

C. Delivery of Care Method
1. The method of delivering patient care on 8 West is consistent with the goals and philosophy of the department of nursing.
2. See Addendum H for policies addressing the following issues:
   a. Delivery of care method,
   b. RN responsibilities,
   c. Assignments,
   d. Reports,
   e. Charge nurse,
   f. Responsibilities of non-professional staff.
3. See Addendum E for a unit diagram of the nursing teams.


D. PREPARATION

This final subsection of your staffing policies addresses those issues related to hiring, orientation, education and validating competency. Here you'll need to define your approaches to the following topics in the preparation of nurses for staff work:

Selection:
How are nurses selected for assignment to your unit? What qualifications must they have? How are interviews conducted? Are job descriptions and performance standards shared with applicants during the interview? What would you consider a serious limitation for an applicant? What options do you have for deal-

ing with new graduates, "refresher" nurses, or nurses with little recent experience?

Orientation and special preparation:

How do you generally orient new staff members to your department? Specifically, how do you prepare new staff members to work independently on your nursing unit? How do you orient them to your expectations of knowledge and skill levels? To your unit standards? How long does this last? Do you use a preceptor program or "buddy" system? How and when are orientees evaluated?

Continuing education:

What are you doing to provide continuing education for your staff? How is your staff development program related to quality assurance activities? How do you provide for mandatory reviews of CPR-readiness, infection control, and safety issues, as required by JCAH? What responsibilities must a staff member assume for staff development? Are staff expected to participate in periodic self evaluation? In QA activities? What are the obligations of the institution? Do your mandate certain topics or contact hours? How do you document your educational activities?

Credentialing:

What are you doing to certify or validate that your staff is competent and meets required knowledge and skill levels? How often do you measure competence? How do you determine if staff are properly licensed? The issue of competency needs to be defined through job descriptions and performance standards, maintained through staff development and employee appraisal activities, and finally validated through annual unit based testing. If you test staff, what corrective measures are taken when knowledge or skill limitations are found?

The above points should be summarized in your general policies and the details specified in the addenda. Some of the content of this subsection will change with shifts in administrative style and management philosophy. Remember, too, that many of these will be contract issues where unions are involved.

For example:

D. Preparation
   1. Selection
      a. Staff will be hired for 8 West by the PCS in collaboration with the ADN for medical/surgical areas. Staff will be selected based on current vacancies, education and experience and an interview. (See Addendum I)
   2. Orientation
      a. All 8 West staff will participate in hospital and unit orien-

tation programs which are structured, formalized, and individualized.
3. Continuing Education
    a. All staff will participate in ongoing educational events held within the Department of Nursing and on 8 West. These educational activities will be based on routine and new responsibilities of nursing staff, identified learning needs, and data from patient care review activities.
4. Credentialing
    a. All staff will be expected to participate in periodic methods to determine learning needs including surveys, questionnaires, and unsolicited suggestions for continuing education events.

## IX. NURSING RESPONSIBILITIES

This final element completes your unit's structure standards. It focuses on identifying responsibilities of your nursing staff with regard to patient care. This section literally lists and discusses what activities each staff group—RN's and LPN's—is allowed to do. It gives the staff members permission to act in certain critical situations, specifically defines their boundaries of function, and limits what physicians can "order" nurses to do. The focus here is on three questions:

- What controversial care measures are nurses allowed to do?
- What high risk measures are staff members allowed to implement?
- What confusing aspects of function by the staff must be clarified?

Finally, this section provides the basis for the writing of process standards in the format of job descriptions and performance standards. Here is an important distinction: Your policies "authorize" staff to act; job descriptions and performance standards outline expectations for function. Remember the hierarchy: **Structure** provides the basis for **Process. Permission** to act must precede **expectations** to act.

This section must address certain JCAH requirements in the areas of Responsibility for:

- using the nursing process,
- keeping the doctor informed of significant changes in a patient's status,
- handling emergency situations,
- performing procedures that put the patient or staff member at risk (not common medical/surgical procedures that all RN's typically perform),
- use of standing orders.

In defining nursing responsibilities, the generic department of nursing policies will outline what all nurses are allowed to do. Your unit specific policies need only address those issues which are relevant to your patient population. Usually the statements are written in a positive manner, or what nurses can do.

However, the statements could be written in the negative, or what nurses are not allowed to do. Be as specific as possible and address RN's and LPN's separately. For example, are nurses in Labor and Delivery allowed to perform rectal and vaginal exams or to treat fetal distress observed on a fetal monitor? Could an RN in orthopaedics cut a cast if she observes seriously impaired circulation in an extremity? Could a psych nurse place a patient in restraints or seclusion before she has an order if the patient is a threat to self or others? Can a nurse reinsert a tracheostomy if the patient pulls it out? Can oncology nurses give experimental drugs?

If you work in a critical care area, you must spell out responsibilities in relation to carrying out "standing emergency orders". Clarify what level of personnel can perform procedures such as defibrillation, IV push of emergency drugs, intubation, cardioversion, and so forth. Also specify what level of training and supervision is required for these activities to take place.

Many of the responsibilities nurses now carry can be traced back to one of serveral scenarios. Perhaps doctors once had a particular responsibility, but they don't feel like using it anymore, so they've delegated it to nursing. Some of these responsibilities are far from trivial matters—manipulating intracardiac lines, for example, or pronouncing patients dead. Perhaps the system provides for someone other than a nurse to carry out the task but, for one reason or another, this arrangement has turned out to be neither practical nor cost-effective, so nursing has taken it over. Examples that come readily to mind are drawing blood for arterial blood gas analysis—because it's faster if a nurse does it—and intubating patients—because no one else ever seems to be around to do it.

Perhaps nurses are offered the opportunity to expand their role by doing things they have never been allowed to do before. Because these new responsibilities fulfill certain psychological needs, the nursing staff embraces them even at the cost of greater workloads and abdication of more traditional nursing responsibilities.

What we define as nursing responsibilities must first fit into our value system, our definition of the role of a professional nurse, with the goal of meeting the needs of doctors and the system considered secondarily. At least six points should be considered in determining what constitutes nursing responsibilities:

1. Is the act in question legal? Is it consistent with the state's Nurse Practice Act?
2. Is it consistent with community standards? (Collecting data about what nurses in area hospitals are doing might help you decide what approach to take.)
3. Is it defined by hospital, department, division, or unit structure as a nursing responsibility?
4. Is there a process standard to outline the nursing function or patient care involved in the activity? In other words, if the action is psychomotor skill, is there an existing procedure? If the action involves a care management situation, is there an existing protocol?
5. If the responsibility has been delegated by a doctor, has the nurse

obtained a doctor's order to do the task now for this particular patient?

6. Finally, is the nurse competent to do the job?

The following examples of nursing responsibilities show how these policies should be written. They might not necessarily be the same responsibilities you'll want to spell out for your unit, but they'll give you some ideas to work with. Note that three categories of function are included: general, psychomotor skill, and emergency measures.

For example:

IX. NURSING RESPONSIBILITIES
  A. The professional staff on 8 West has these responsibilities:
    1. General:
       a. All those responsibilities listed in generic department of nursing policies including the use of the nursing process when giving patient care.
       b. Knowledge and use of physical and psychosocial assessment skills as specified in the units performance standards.
    2. Psychomotor skills:
       a. Administering IV push and continuous drip medications, as specified in department of nursing policy.
       b. Starting peripheral IV lines with physician's order.
    3. Emergency measures:
       a. Performing CPR as specified by the Resuscitation Committee.
       b. Implementing emergency protocols, as specified in the unit's standards manual, assuming the staff member has been approved and is recertified annually.

More extensive examples of policies governing staffing and nursing responsibilities can be found in the Sample Unit Standards Manual.

Now that your policies are complete, you're ready to move to writing process standards—building upon the foundation you've erected with structure standards.

# UNIT III PROCESS STANDARDS:

## Adding Substance

Process standards define the actions and behaviors expected of staff as well as what constitutes safe and effective patient care. They are action-oriented and directed at either the NURSE or the PATIENT. Your process standards are likely to be quite extensive as they encompass everything that nurses know, do, and believe. They are based on the nursing process.

You'll recall from Chapter Two, Process Standards can be written in six formats:

- Job Descriptions
- Performance Standards
- Procedures
- Protocols
- Guidelines
- Standards of Care

In this unit, we will examine each format, discussing its style or layout, appropriate content, and writing technique. Once you have decided the style of a particular format, staff can readily "fill in the blanks" with content. The drafted standard will then be ready for approval, education, implementation, and monitoring follow-up.

# Chapter 8   Job Descriptions and Performance Standards

Job descriptions are an excellent starting point for defining what you expect of employees. This format outlines general duties and responsibilities for a level of worker. It serves as a basis for hiring, for delineating employee qualifications, and for substantiating the institution's commitment to those legal, regulatory, and professional standards to which it is accountable.

The Job Description is a broad overview of a person's work. It is directed at a level or classification of worker—a person who meets specific qualifications, is hired to perform certain activities, and paid accordingly. This means that there should be *only one* job description for each level of worker: staff RNs, LPNs, head nurses, nursing assistants, clinical specialists, staff development instructors, nursing office supervisors, and so forth, regardless of the number of persons filling that category of employee.

## ORIGIN AND CONTENT

Where do job descriptions originate? Most evolve within the institution from management's interpretation of legal definitions of practice, JCAH and state requirements, and existing professional standards. For example, the job description of a staff RN reflects her state nurse practice act, JCAH Nursing Service Standards, and ANA practice standards. The common thread running through all three origins is the nursing process. Thus all staff nurse job descriptions must include this as a major professional responsibility. While the nursing process reflects the staff nurse's direct patient care duties, she also has numerous other responsibilities. Table 8-1 lists twenty-eight (28) activities that constitute the role of the staff RN around which her job description should be developed. The activities are divided into categories of nursing process, professionalism, growth and staff development, and leadership and coordination.

## TABLE 8-1

## Activities of Staff RN

| **NURSING PROCESS** |
| --- |

1. Assessment.
2. Use of nursing diagnosis.
3. Goal setting.
4. Planning.
5. Implementation (dependent and independent actions).
6. Evaluation.
7. Technical competency.
8. Patient/family education.
9. Concern for patient/family rights.
10. Safety.
11. Emergency situations.
12. Knowledge base and use of standards in patient care.

| **PROFESSIONALISM, GROWTH AND DEVELOPMENT** |
| --- |

13. Responsibility/accountability for own practice (including appearance, attendance, and punctuality).
14. Participation in staff development activities for other staff.
15. Participation in self directed learning and continuing education for self.
16. Seeking guidance/validation when necessary.
17. Legal issues.
18. Attainment of unit/department goals.
19. Participation in peer review and quality assurance activities.
20. Flexibility in 24 hour scheduling practices.
21. Participation in research activities.

| **LEADERSHIP AND COORDINATION** |
| --- |

22. Delegation and direction of others.
23. Communication.
24. Working relationships.
25. Coordination and organization.
26. Priority setting abilities.
27. Use of lines of authority.
28. Problem solving abilities.

In consideration of the job description for a nurse manager, Table 8-2 lists twenty-two (22) activities that constitute the role of the first line manager (head nurse, nurse manager, nurse coordinator, patient care supervisor, or whatever the title may be) around which the job description should be developed. It includes both clinical and managerial responsibilities as well as those identified by JCAH in the Nursing Service Standards.

TABLE 8-2

## Activities of Nurse Manager

1. Clinical expertise.
2. Role modeling and clinical direction.
3. Nursing process.
4. Safety issues.
5. Budgetary activities.
6. Legal issues.
7. Committee work and meetings.
8. Policy development.
9. Standards (other than structure).
10. JCAH responsibilities
11. Quality assurance.
12. Appraisal of employees.
13. Licensure.
14. Hiring.
15. Staff development.
16. Staffing.
17. Self growth and development.
18. Communication.
19. Working relationships.
20. Leadership.
21. Problem solving.
22. Nursing research.

## BUILDING THE JOB DESCRIPTION

Building a job description is not a difficult task. It really should take no more than a few hours if you focus on three points. First, keep it simple and brief—no more than one or two pages. Remember that it is an overview only. Second, direct it at a category of worker such as staff RN's, not individuals within a category such as an ICU nurse or a medical surgical RN. Third, include the necessary components of a job description and adhere to content within each component. There are seven (7) components to the job description, the second of which is optional:

1. TITLE.
2. IDENTIFICATION (optional).
3. JOB SUMMARY.
4. STATEMENT OF ACCOUNTABILITY.
5. GENERAL DUTIES AND RESPONSIBILITIES.
6. QUALIFICATIONS.
7. APPROVAL.

The title should state what the tool is to be called and the category of worker for which it is written. Different systems choose various titles such as job description, position description, position profile, position summary, and so forth. Here, the document is the traditional job description with the level of worker proceeding the title: "Staff Nurse (RN) Job Description" or "Head Nurse Job Description."

The second component, identification, consists of personnel data such as hours to be worked per pay period, weekend responsibilities, salary status (hourly, exempt, non-exempt), employee department title or number, and so forth. Since this is generally considered to be position control information and is found on computer printouts, it is optional and may be eliminated from the job description *per se*. Of course, this information would still be discussed with the applicant at the interview.

Next, the job description should include a job summary. This brief paragraph describes the primary function of the level of worker. It is also referred to as basic function, main responsibility, or position summary. Regardless, it gives the job description its focus and should not include specific tasks.

For example:

JOB SUMMARY: The staff RN is a professional care giver who assumes reponsibility and accountability for a group of patients for a designated time frame and provides care to these patients via therapeutic use of self, the nursing process, the environment/instrumentation, and other health care team members.

Following this, is a statement that identifies the accountability of the employee. This may be called "reports to" or "accountable to" or "immediate superior." Because of its importance, this statement should stand alone and not be incorporated into the job summary.

For example:

REPORTS TO: Head Nurse of unit to which assigned.
Next is the bulk of the job description, the general duties and responsibilities. These are behavioral statements, beginning with an action verb such as demonstrates, functions, performs, participates, formulates, and so forth. Identify key functions of the work and write one statement to reflect the required behavior. Do not elaborate with specific details. This is not the tool for it. The job description should appear as a list, not an outline with multiple sub-

divisions. In relation to content, be comprehensive and include all functions of the position. For example, in the head nurse job description, don't just speak to management duties, but address both clinical and management functions. Refer back to the lists of 28 activities of the staff RN and 22 activities of the head nurse. It is acceptable to combine two like areas such as legal and safety issues. It is helpful to write the areas of function using one or two words to the left hand side of the statements. This allows the reader to quickly scan the job description for a particular piece of information. An example for a nurse manager might read:

*POLICY:*      8. Follows Hospital and Departmental policies, participates in their development and uses them as a basis for decision making for both clinical and management issues.

*STANDARDS:* 9. Participates in the development of criteria based job descriptions as directed and in the writing of performance standards for employees in her area.

Qualifications for the job should cover three areas of requirements: education and credentials, experience, and physical attributes.

For example:

QUALIFICATIONS:
1. Current State License.
2. BSN required.
3. Documented experience and expertise in clinical area relevant to unit patient population (minimum of 3-5 years clinical work).
4. Documented experience and expertise in management area either in first line or shift supervisory work.
5. Excellent physical, communication, and writing abilities.

Finally, the job description should reflect dates and mechanisms (persons or group) of approval followed by review and revision dates. The review date tells when the tool will be updated, the revision when last updated.

## LIMITATIONS OF JOB DESCRIPTIONS

Despite the importance of the job description, this format has three serious limitations. It simply is not specific enough to define the precise performance expectations, knowledge base, and psychomotor skills required by a nurse working on a particular unit. Consider these examples.

*Prepares discharge plans for all patients assigned to her care.*

Medical/surgical nurse: "I must attend discharge rounds and discuss implications for my patients at home or the need for extended custodial care."

ICU nurse: "My patients are transferred to another unit, so this part of the job description must not apply to me."

| Psych unit nurse: | "I must plan for the outpatient therapy, based on community resources, or decide that certain patients need long-term hospitalization." |

*Performs general nursing procedures according to established protocols.*

| Medical/surgical nurse: | "I must know how to change dressings, hang IV's, administer medications, and take care of tubes and catheters." |
| ICU nurse: | "I must know how to monitor arterial lines, interpret arrhythmias, care for intubated patients on ventilators, give IV medications, and manage intracardiac lines." |
| Psych unit nurse: | "I must know how to conduct community meetings, follow a consistent therapeutic approach, and provide a controlled milieu." |

*Demonstrates priority setting abilities.*

| Medical/surgical nurse: | "My assignments are fair and equal for my team, emergency needs of patients are met, routine care is provided and documented, and everybody finishes their shift on time." |
| ICU nurse: | "Nursing care is provided in conjunction with ongoing medical management; my patient has uninterrupted rest periods, but all nursing procedures and medical treatments are completed as ordered." |
| Psych unit nurse: | "Meetings and therapeutic sessions are conducted as scheduled; patients receive occupational, art, and music therapy as planned." |

As these situations demonstrate, the nurse who works on medical/surgical unit doesn't function the same as the ICU or psych unit nurse. The job description, by its very nature, generalizes and provides a common definition of function for all nurses. To differentiate among nurses who take care of different types of patients requires more detail.

The job description is also inadequate to promote progressive development of the worker. Developing staff members effectively requires determining a nurse's **current** level of performance and comparing it to a **desired** level of performance; then both you and the staff member can plan how to reach the desired level through clearly defined expectations. Generic job descriptions are too vague to let you do that.

Finally, the job description alone, won't permit an effective evaluation. While a job description is the traditional vehicle for performance appraisal, it lacks the specificity you need to judge staff function at the unit level. This basic inadequacy compromises both the manager, who may agonize over evaluations, using such a nonspecific tool, and the staff nurse, who may be an expert critical care practitioner with 20 years experience, but who is still evaluated by the same general job description as a new medical-surgical nurse.

The answer to this dilemma is to extend job descriptions into Performance standards.

## THE VITAL LINK

Performance standards define the level of practice required to maintain the desired quality of nursing care. The key words in this definition are "the level of practice required." Performance standards serve as the vital link between staff performance and the care required by a patient population on a unit. In any nursing system, all RN's are expected to perform according to their job description, but the specific definition, interpretation, and application of its content must be incorporated into performance standards.

Don't get confused over terms here. JCAH surveyors frequently refer to "standards of practice," but that's a rather vague term, whereas "performance standards" is more specific. Both terms, however, refer to the same thing—defining management's expectations for employees!

Performance standards don't exist in isolation, but grow out of the underlying job description. In other words, nothing can be written into performance standards which the job description does not address. Expectations of staff evolve in response to the work setting. So while all RNs in a nursing system assess, plan, document, and communicate, only performance standards can define precisely how a nurse working on a particular unit would go about accomplishing these activities. Nurses working in labor and delivery unit, for example, assess their patients and use monitoring devices; the same is true of nurses working in a coronary care unit. Performance standards are needed to define how each group of nurses would assess their different patient populations. In the case of labor and delivery nurses, their performance standards for assessment would address vaginal and rectal exams and fetal monitoring, while those written for the CCU nurses would deal with identifying heart sounds and friction rubs or invasive hemodynamic pressure monitoring.

Performance standards are also directed at the average acuity level of patients in an area. The myocardial infarction patient needs a competent ER nurse to assess and treat his pain and potentially life-threatening arrhythmias and heart failure. When this patient arrives in the CCU, the nurses there will have the same concerns as the ER nurses, but they'll place more emphasis on his psychological and cognitive needs because these will become more evident as his physiologic status stabilizes. Once this same patient is transferred to the step-down unit, the nurses there will be concerned about preparing him for self care and discharge. Thus the patient's changing acuity level influences the care he'll require, in turn influencing what nurses need to know, be, and do. Performance standards are designed to elucidate precisely these varied levels of function, knowledge and skill.

Finally, performance standards reflect the nursing values of the unit leaders. Nurse managers have different interpretations of what constitutes good performance. Because the first-line manager is involved in interviewing, hiring, supervising, and evaluating her staff, she should also be involved in defining expectations. Thus, performance standards are written:

- for a specific patient population on a specific unit (or common units within the system);
- in relation to the acuity level of the patient population;
- in the context of the values of nursing leadership.

## USING PERFORMANCE STANDARDS

Performance standards can prove invaluable in several different aspects of management:

- Selection: Use the job description and your performance standards when you interview a prospective employee. Does this person's experience and education meet your expectations? Share the job description and unit specific performance standards with the applicant. Are they acceptable to her? If so, then you have two sound reasons for hiring: The applicant meets the requirements for the position and can probably adjust to your unit.
- Orientation: Establish the level of performance expected of a new staff member as soon as he/she starts working on the unit. Performance standards can be very useful here—orienting the new employee to what the rest of the staff does and what is expected of them. If orientation is based on specific performance standards, you're more likely to have a competent, independent practitioner working for you at the end of this adjustment period.
- Development: Performance standards can promote development of staff members by defining what constitutes efficient performance. This allows you to examine staff members in relation to established standards. You can thus identify deficiencies more readily and plan pertinent continuing education events to improve performance and move the staff toward a higher level of practice. Performance standards can also help you justify the time and money spent on staff development. Ultimately, your staff development sessions should be directed either to maintaining staff competency defined in performance standards or to assisting staff to respond to new competencies added to the unit's performance standards.
- Supervision: Performance standards can serve as the basis for your supervisory activities. Use them when you make rounds or interact with staff in any coaching session. You might have to keep them in your pocket or on a clip board until everyone gets used to them! Often staff members need time to adjust to such specifically defined expectations. Use your performance standards to provide feedback to the staff in both verbal and written form. Written expectations are the basis for excellent anecdotal records to monitor staff performance throughout the year.
- Evaluation: Using performance standards, you can more effectively evaluate the performance of a worker being considered for promotion, a merit raise, or dismissal. Simply incorporate your performance standards into your current appraisal system. Evaluate your staff by their common job description and your unit specific performance standards. In fact, their ability to carry out the unit performance standards is the basis for their final rating in relation to the job description behaviors.

# AVOIDING PITFALLS IN DEVELOPING
# PERFORMANCE STANDARDS

**Unit Versus Division.** Remember that performance standards are patient population and unit specific. Each unit needs its own set of performance standards to define the functions and scope of practice of its staff, such as 5 North (Orthopedics) or 6 South (Oncology) or Operating Room. If however, a system is set up so that several units have similar patients and their staffs function in basically the same manner, then only one set of performance standards needs to be written for the entire division. Just as with structure standards, ask yourself "Am I more alike or more different than my sister units?" If you are very different, write unit based performance standards (ICU, CCU, OR, PAR, ER, PSYCHIATRY, LABOR AND DELIVERY, POST PARTUM, PEDIATRICS). If you are similar to other units, write performance standards aimed at all the common units or division based performance standards (Medical Division, Surgical Division, Special Care Division, Ambulatory Care Division). If you choose the division approach, a set of the performance standards would still appear in each unit's standards manual.

**Who should write them?** Performance standards should be written by all levels of managers with assistance from the staff members they supervise. Because expectations are generally established by the superior for the subordinate, the director of nursing should write performance standards for assistant directors, the assistant directors for head nurses, and the head nurse for her staff. Of course, this should be a participative activity, but the person ultimately responsible for defining expectations and boundaries of function remains that of the superior. It is inappropriate to dump this responsibility casually and call it delegation unless the superior simultaneously provides solid direction and guidance. On the other hand, to autocratically adopt performance standards that are unacceptable to one's subordinates is foolish. Thus once the performance standards are written in draft form, they should be shared with staff members for feedback on content. The manager may accept or reject suggestions for additions, deletions, or modifications, but she should see to it that her staff is given the opportunity to provide input.

**Generic Versus Specific.** With the job description as the basis for staff function, you have another decision to make. You can write performance standards which are generic for the entire department of nursing and then write those for the unit/division. Or you may elect to omit the generic work and go from the job description straight to unit/division specific performance standards.

The former approach appeals to some managers by providing a common base for unit specific performance standards. However, it requires extra writing time and delays the completion of the essential unit performance standards. You may skip this intermediate step and devote your attention to the more critical definition of expectations at the unit level.

**Career Ladders and Performance Standards.** The issue of generic performance standards raises two serious questions about career ladders and performance standards. First, if your system uses a career ladder, don't be fooled into thinking that you have (or require) more than one RN job description. For example, let's say you've developed three classifications of progressive performance for your RN's—Staff Nurse I, II, and III. You wouldn't want to label the definitions of these classifications "job descriptions" because, of course, they are not. There is still only one job description for all staff RN's in the system. The definition of Staff Nurse I, II, and III should be considered generic performance standards because they apply to all units. The second problem is that the career ladder typically is generic and falls short of unit based performance standards. This work still remains to be done. For example, CCU, ER, and 5 North (Orthopedics) may have Staff Nurse I's, II's, and III's working in each area. But what are the precise expectation in relation to the patient populations, acuity, and leadership values? Regardless of how many "levels" a career ladder has, unit based performance standards for each level and on each unit must still be written. Here again, to skip the generic career ladder phase and develop specific measurable performance standards at the unit level is preferable.

## WRITING PERFORMANCE STANDARDS

Essentially, writing performance standards requires four steps. First, take the job description and read each statement, making a list of areas in which the worker must perform. Use only one or two words to reflect each work area. For the staff RN, the list might look something like this:

*STEP 1:*

- assessment
- nursing diagnosis
- goal setting
- care planning
- implementation
- communication
- patient teaching
- growth and development
- working relationships
- dealing with emergencies
- professional behaviors
- documentation

Second, make two columns—one called "Priority I Behaviors" and the other "Priority II Behaviors". Take another look at your original list of work areas and divide the items between these two columns. While you might consider all the areas important, chances are some are more critical to you and your patients than others. This ranking will develop your most important performance standards first and address others later. Eventually you will want to have a complete set for all areas in the job description. Your priority lists might look like this:

*STEP 2:*

| *PRIORITY I BEHAVIORS* | *PRIORITY II BEHAVIORS* |
|---|---|
| • assessment | • communication |
| • nursing diagnosis | • patient teaching |
| • care planning | • growth and development |
| • implementation | • working relationships |
| • emergency situations | • professional behavior |
| • documentation | |

Third, take your priority I behavior areas and decide what each one means to you. Expand the word or phrase you've chosen to describe each of these aspects of a staff nurse's job into some specific behaviors or actions that would be exhibited by the ideal employee. Don't strain for specifics here. Just "brainstorm" what each word or phrase reflects in the way of quality performance. Jot down any ideas that come to mind. You might want to ask yourself questions, then write down the answers in general terms. For example:

*STEP 3:*

ASSESSMENT:
What parameters constitute assessment on the unit?
Who is responsible for performing assessment?
How does assessment differ from observation?
How often is assessment performed during a shift or patient stay?
When does an assessment occur?
How will the assessment be recorded? Within what time frames?

As you reflect on the answers to such questions, you should begin to get some firm ideas about what assessment includes; whether you require a systems approach or a head-to-toe method; what differentiates RN assessment activities from LPN observation tasks; when assessment should take place on admission, during the shift, at transfer and discharge; where assessment information is to be documented and when. After Step 3, your worksheet might include:

ASSESSMENT:

What parameters constitute assessment on this unit?
> Systems
> Head to toe
> Neuro
> CV/Pulmonary
> GU/GI
> M/S/Integ

Who is responsible for performing assessment?
> Admission RN
> Assigned RN for shift

How does assessment differ from observation?

> data collection
> analysis
> action LPN
> data collection only
> reporting requiring validation for
> interpretation

When does assessment occur?

> Admission into unit
> Transfer to unit
> Discharge from unit
> During each shift
> Expiration

How often is assessment performed during a shift or patient stay?

> Early in shift (2 hours)
> Repeated
> Midpoint
> End of shift

How will the assessment be recorded? Within what time frame?

> Initial on NDB
> (Nursing Data Base)
> within 24 hours
> Each Shift on Unit
> AFS (Assessment Flow
> Sheet) within 2 hours

Finally, after your worksheet is filled with notes from brainstorming, you are ready to translate each idea into performance standards. Make each performance expectation as specific and measurable as possible. Follow the assessment example through these steps and your final performance standards might look like this:

1. Assessment
   a. Performs admission assessment on all patients admitted within *24 hours* on NDB per guidelines.
   b. If initial admission on another unit, reviews this as baseline and completes unit assessment *within 20 minutes* after arrival of patient.
   c. Performs shift assessment *within 2 hours* of coming on duty. Includes:

   NEURO: LOC/mental status/orientation/psychological attitude
   CV: Skin warmth/color
   rate/respiration/BP
   Neck veins @45
   PUL: Breathing patterns
   Ant./post. chest sounds

GU/GI:      Abdominal flatness, softness, BS, flatus/
            BM/Urine qs/color/method
MS/INTEG:   ROM adequacy
            Wound/dressing/tube condition/drainage IV
            site/condition/infusion status
            Skin condition (dependent areas for lesions/edema)

d. *Repeats shift assessment mid-point and end of shift* with focus on organ/system of pathology.
e. Performs shift assessment at transfer or discharge from unit.
f. Documents shift assessment on unit assessment flowsheet *within 2 hours* of coming on duty and *mid-point and end of shift* according to form guidelines.

## IMPLEMENTATION

One last important point about performance standards. Don't expect to include all your expectations of staff members in the first set of performance standards you write. Give them time to change and grow as you become more experienced at using them. Try your first set of standards for six months to a year. See how well they serve your needs; keep notes of things that need to be added. Daily interactions with your staff will provide plenty of ideas for future performance standards. Eventually you will refine your performance standards to truly reflect your expectations of the people you supervise.

After you've written your performance standards read them over carefully, noting their degree of specificity and measurability. You're now ready to share them with your staff. Small group review sessions should suffice for clarifying content and validating staff's understanding of the meaning and use of performance standards. Consider their suggestions for any modifications, then set a target date for implementing the expectations. Implementation means using the performance standards in your nursing system as a basis for employee selection, orientation, daily supervision, employee performance monitoring through anecdotal records, and employee appraisal as previously discussed.

Samples of RN performance standards appear in the Unit Standards Manual.

# Chapter 9:  Procedures and Protocols

## PROCEDURES

Procedures are step by step instructions on how to perform psychomotor skills. They concern nursing tasks specifically and have both a technical and theoretical basis. The **technical** portion gives precise directions on getting the task done and should be limited to "how to":

- insert and remove invasive devices.
- attach and disconnect equipment.
- administer and discontinue medical treatments.
- perform nursing actions for physical testing/assessment or intervention.

The following is a brief list of common nursing procedures. Note the task focus and how each topic fits into one of the above four categories.

- Insert a salem sump/feeding tube.
- Irrigate a Foley catheter.
- Assist with inserting a subclavian line.
- Measure central venous pressure.
- Insert a heparin lock.
- Set-up and administer hyperalimentation.
- Change renal shunt dressing.
- Change a pacemaker dressing.
- Irrigate a colostomy.
- Administer tube feedings.
- Change an established trach tube.
- Suction endotrachially (with an artificial airway in place).
- Assist with bronchoscopy.
- Assist with insertion of chest tubes and set-up drainage container.
- Perform a vaginal exam on a laboring patient.
- Set-up and attach a fetal monitor.

The **theoretical** basis for a procedure usually involves the scientific and nursing rationales for certain actions. When carefully worded, it adds credence and sophistication to those actions and should focus on safety factors to minimize risk to both the nurse and patient. The theoretical basis must be supportive to the procedure steps and not dominate the procedure or add unnecessary length.

Procedures can be written to reflect various levels of nursing skills. Obviously, some procedures are strictly nursing tasks which the nurse can independently decide to perform and do so alone, such as oral hygiene, passive range-of-motion, and fractional urines. Other procedures can be carried out by the nurse but only after being ordered by the physician. Examples would be administering medications, inserting a Foley catheter, and starting a tube feeding. Still other procedures are entirely dependent, requiring the nurse to assist the doctor in some task, such as inserting a central venous line or performing a bedside bronchoscopy. Finally, performing some procedures is controversial for the nurse and her ability to do so is governed by the institution. Examples of these procedures include endotracheal suctioning, changing trachs and surgical dressings, irrigating IVs and drainage tubes, inserting artificial airways, and performing emergency measures such as defibrillation. Obviously, since nursing skills can be defined at different levels, structure standards (policies) for the department of nursing and each unit must clearly specify what staff is allowed to do under "nursing responsibilities." The procedure itself might reiterate this information. However, the procedure does not give the nurse permission to perform—structure standards do that. The procedure merely explains how to do the task described.

Procedures can also be categorized by their application. **Generic** procedures are those performed by all nurses on all units; **Specific** procedures are performed only by certain nurses on designated units. The advantage of this separation is that it allows you to put generic procedures in a Generic Department of Nursing Standards Manual available on all units, while housing specific procedures in unit or division based standards manuals only where they apply. This prevents unnecessary duplication of effort, reduces volume of information not relevant to certain staff members, and makes locating a particular procedure easier. Because each procedure will contain a distribution list as a component, this segregation is easily accomplished. Staff can readily differentiate which tasks are special for their area from those which apply to all units.

### Common Problems

There are three serious problems commonly associated with the current writing of nursing procedures.

1. *Too many procedures.* While there should be a written procedure for every psychomotor skill performed by nurses, some method should limit the number to 100 or less. The limit prevents staff from feeling overwhelmed when trying to locate a particular procedure. There are three easy ways to accomplish this. First, critique your procedures and remove any topic that is not a psychomotor skill. Second, separate the procedures into generic (applicable to all units) and specific (applicable to certain units only). Third, combine like topics into one procedure. For

example, instead of writing separate procedures on apical rates, blood pressure, and electronic temperature recording, combine all into one procedure on "Vital Signs Recording." Instead of writing separate procedures on inserting a CVP, changing the tubing, changing the dressing, recording the CVP, discontinuing the line, combine all the relevant issues into one procedure. This strategy decreases the overall number of procedures eliminating repetition and wasted space, and contributes to ease of use.

2. *Insufficient quality:* All procedures serve an educational purpose. Information and directions presented must be relevant, accurate, and current. To be effective, your procedures must not only be easy to find but quick to use. When a nurse refers to a procedure she needs to be able to scan it rapidly for needed information and visually validate essential issues such as necessary supplies, connection of equipment, and potential pitfalls.

   Important quality considerations include adopting a consistent style, controlling length, and including extensive illustration. Obviously, selecting a **consistent style** contributes uniformity to procedures written by staff in different clinical areas. Proper sequencing of steps, sufficient detailed content to prevent assumption, and using two columns for content are all important measures designed to make the procedure easy to read and use. **Controlling length** is important because of the total number of procedures required in a nursing system. Generally, you should try to keep your procedures to one to two pages each (front and back). This should not be difficult if wording is precise, rationale kept at a minimum, and space on the paper is maximized. The exception to the one to two page rule is, of course, when you combine several tasks into one procedure. These "combined" procedures are often three to four pages in length (front and back). Finally, improve readability and shorten overall length by freely illustrating your procedures. Drawings, diagrams, or photocopied illustrations from equipment inserts and texts add visual emphasis and can effectively take the place of extra words.

3. *Inappropriate Content:* The traditional approach to writing procedures has created the current situation of "Procedure Abuse." Inserting information not related to performing a psychomotor skill has added unnecessary length and complexity to procedures. Lengthy, complicated tools do not get used.

   The nursing procedure should not contain "nursing management." Controlling length is only one reason. There are two others. First, philosophically, psychomotor skills comprise only a small—but important—aspect of professional nursing practice. Many skills are delegated to other personnel such as LPNs, nursing assistants, and technicians. While tasks may easily be assigned, the nursing management associated with the tasks often cannot. For example, an RN delegates the task of assisting a physician with a bedside insertion on a chest tube to an LPN. This is fine, assuming the LPN has been properly trained. However, the care and management of this therapy involving critical assessments, interventions for complications, and decision making for effective functioning remain ultimately the responsibility of the RN. While this is not to say that an LPN cannot care for a patient with a chest tube, note that tasks and skills are different from knowledge, decision making, and use of nursing process—and that the former can be delegated but the latter cannot. Therefore, if we lump everything together—tasks and higher level nursing practice—the ability to differentiate between professional nursing and ancillary assistance becomes more and more difficult.

Second, from a practical standpoint, nurses refer to procedures when they need to know "how to" do something. New employees and new graduates use procedures quite often. However, veteran staff seldom rely on procedures because they are secure in their psychomotor abilities. Thus, if your procedures confuse tasks and ongoing nursing care and many of your nurses do not refer to them because they no longer require technical assistance, the nursing management content will "be out of sight and out of mind" and unavailable for implementation. Your own unit QA activities probably show that psychomotor tasks are followed more consistently than higher level care and management interventions.

Let's pursue our chest tube example. Your procedure on "Chest Tubes" should address the following issues relating to assisting with insertion:

- gathering the equipment needed,
- preparing the patient,
- preparing the wound site,
- setting up a sterile field,
- handing equipment to the physician,
- preparing and connecting the chest drainage system,
- applying a dressing.

In addition, it should combine other task oriented measures such as changing the drainage system, aspirating a sample, and discontinuing the tube. But of course the nurse's responsibilities do not end with the insertion and associated tasks involving the chest tube. As a matter of fact, you could say the professional care is just beginning after the tube is in place. Consider the following:

- patient positioning to promote lung expansion and drainage,
- time frames for altering this position,
- routine for performing chest assessment (parameters and frequency)
- information to be reported to the physician,
- care of the chest tube (maintaining water level, stripping frequency and evaluation, checking for air leaks),
- wound and dressing care (assessment, reinforcement, or dressing change),
- pain management (whether to medicate before or after activity, pain assessment, supportive measures to minimize discomfort),
- hydration issues (use of intake and output, marking the drainage and container),

- pulmonary care (use of suctioning, postural drainage and chest physical therapy),
- bedside supplies (proximity of extra drainage containers, lubricated gauze, connectors, rubber-shod clamps and when to use the clamps),
- emergency nursing functions (accidental dislodgement of the tube or disconnection, container reaches maximum capacity, occlusion of the drainage tube).

These issues are not simple nursing tasks; they have nothing to do with the insertion of the chest tube and do not belong in your procedure on "Chest Tubes." These issues are more complex, go on for a defined period of time, and address more sophisticated nursing functions including all aspects of the nursing process and decision making. They are properly defined in the format we'll be discussing later in this chapter—PROTOCOLS. By separating this content, your procedures can be kept simple, to the point, focused on the nurse, and limited to psychomotor skills.

### Recommended Style

A well-written procedure includes these nine components:

- *TITLE:*      Be as complete as possible and use the word "Procedure" to differentiate from other process formats—"Procedure for Assisting Physicians with Bronchoscopy" not just "Bronchoscopy."

- *PURPOSE:*      Be clear—the purpose of any procedure is always to direct the nurse to *do* something safely and efficiently. This should be limited to a single sentence.

|  | | | |
|---|---|---|---|
| TO | • delineate | NURSING | • methodology   IN: |
|  | • specify | | • responsibility |
|  | • define | | • role |
|  | • outline | | |

- *SUPPORTIVE DATA:* Provide information necessary to the nurse in carrying out the task, such as indications, definitions, physician responsibilities, who may perform task, purpose of equipment. Be as brief as possible. Limit: a paragraph. Use this section to cross-reference the procedure to a corresponding protocol.

- *EQUIPMENT LIST:* Include location of equipment off the unit. If this is more than four or five items, use double columns to reduce the length of space needed.

- *CONTENT:*      Place in two-columns, titling the left hand column "Steps" and the right hand column "Key Points." "Key Points" is preferable to "rationale" because it implies that content is limited to essential safety information.

For example:

| STEPS | KEY POINTS |
|---|---|
| • Define detailed, sequential steps of how to proceed. | • Focus on reducing risk to nurse and patient. |
| • Do not make assumptions—spell it out!!! | • Provide cautions to prevent errors common to task. |
| • Number all steps. | |
| • Illustrate and add diagrams to clarify ideas and reduce unnecessary words. | |

- *DOCUMENTATION:* Be specific about what, where, and when charting is to be done.

- *REFERENCE:* Include references. It may be a person or literature but limit to one or two items. May also include the author of the procedure.

- *APPROVAL:* Include original date and mechanism of approval, followed by the review and revision dates.

- *DISTRIBUTION:* Identify whether it is a generic or unit specific procedure and list which nursing units will have it.

An example of the Procedure "Chest Tube Insertion/Drainage Procedure" that illustrates the correct use of all nine style components can be found under Process Standards in the Sample Unit Standards Manual.

### Writing Procedures

Because staff members actually execute the psychomotor skills, they can contribute a great deal to procedure writing. But to delegate the writing of a procedure entirely to a staff nurse without providing adequate direction usually results in disappointment on both sides. That's why adopting a consistent style and incorporating this style into a drafting form is important. A procedure draft should include the nine style components, plus other essential information:

- Name of the institution, department, or unit area (this gives the procedure a professional appearance—never just start writing).
- Drafter's name, draft number, and draft date (this gives the author credit and allows the procedure to be tracked through the approval process).

Using a consistent drafting style allows you to focus your writing on content issues, since style has been determined. The approved final procedure is the final draft. Also, staff nurses using a drafting style are educated in the correct way to write procedures.

With all this information in mind, look critically over your existing procedures. Ask yourself five questions:

1. Have I controlled the overall number of procedures by combining like tasks and differentiating between generic and unit specific tasks?
2. Have I adopted a well planned, consistent style using columns and maximizing space?
3. Have I controlled the length of each procedure by limiting content to essential information, using extensive illustrations, and writing on both sides of the paper?
4. Have I abused the users with inappropriate content which is really best suited to another format?
5. Have I used procedures to address issues which are not related to psychomotor skills?

Your answers to these questions can help you develop better procedures next time they come up for revision. Following the ideas presented in this section can make the difference between procedures that are actively used by the nursing staff and those that gather dust on the shelf.

## PROTOCOLS

Protocols define appropriate nursing action for effective management of common patient care problems. They specify the nursing response to certain patient care issues and establish nursing care routines to ensure quality and continuity. Protocols differ from procedures in that procedures are task-oriented, while protocols relate to ongoing nursing management of patient care problems.

### Categories

Any situation where patient care is given can warrant a protocol. In general, though, protocols can be grouped into five categories:

1. **Managing patients with non-invasive equipment.** Remember, getting the patient on and off the equipment is a psychomotor skill and requires a procedure for proper explanation. But managing the patient while he's on the equipment—whether for 5 minutes or 5 weeks—requires a protocol. Examples of non-invasive equipment requiring protocols in this category include:

   - hypothermia blanket,
   - isolette/croupette,
   - oxygen therapy (care of patient using cannula, catheter, masks),
   - orthopaedic devices (such as traction, casts, pins, halos),
   - medical antishock trousers (MAST),
   - special beds (Stryker frame, circoelectric, and so forth),
   - cardiac monitors (telemetry, hard wire, holter),
   - fetal monitor (external and internal).

Consider the patient on a hypothermia blanket, for example. What content should be addressed when writing the protocol for nursing management of such an issue? Skin protection, especially of extremities? How often should the patient be turned? What special precautions should be taken with high risk patients such as patients with peripheral vascular disease? How often should vital signs be taken, especially temperature? Should the blanket be set on automatic or manual mode? How low can the body temperature be lowered and remain safe? What should be done to keep the patient comfortable? Should he be sedated? What about electrical hazards? What are potential complications and critical interventions for them? How can shivering be controlled? These are the kinds of questions to ask when writing this protocol.

2. **Managing patients with invasive equipment.** Many examples readily come to mind:

   - IV therapy (peripheal and central venous lines),
   - long term venous access (porta-shunts, Hickman lines),
   - umbilical lines,
   - arterial lines (radial, brachial, femoral),
   - ICP lines,
   - intracardiac lines (PA and LA)
   - temporary pacers,
   - chest tubes,
   - GU intubation tubes (indwelling bladder catheters, suprapubic drains, nephrostomy tubes, ureteral catheters, external catheters/leg bags),
   - IABP,
   - external AV shunts,
   - GI intubation tubes (NG, sumps, G-tubes, J-tubes),
   - Blakemore tubes.

3. **Any diagnostic, therapeutic, or prophylactic intervention requiring nursing measures.** Examples include:

   - pre/post biopsy,
   - pre/post cardiac catheterization,
   - pre/post endoscopy,
   - anticoagulant therapy,
   - tube feedings,
   - hyperalimentation,
   - titrated drug therapy (antiarrhythmics, NTG, nitroprusside, streptokinase, pitressin, pitocin, insulin, anticonvulsants, dopamine, aminophylline, psychotropic drugs),
   - peritoneal dialysis,
   - hemofiltration and hemodialysis,
   - chemotherapy,
   - blood products administration,
   - restraints,
   - post electro-convulsive therapy,
   - post cardioversion,
   - routine hygiene/physiologic monitoring (AM/PM care, overhead frames, intake and output, fractional urines, vital signes routines,

hematests, ROM, cradles, sheepskins, heel protectors, vital signs, calorie counts),
- detoxification routines (drugs, ETOH),
- seclusion,
- complicated wound management (special drainage devices, fistulas),
- ostomy care (colostomy, ileostomy).

4. **Physiological or psychological states or conditions.** Examples include:

Physiological:

- preoperative care,
- postoperative management,
- delerium tremors,
- hypoglycemic reaction,
- shock (hypovolemic, cardiogenic, septic, neurogenic),
- seizures,
- post resuscitation care,
- hyperthermia.

Psychological:

- confusion, agitation, wandering,
- suicidal states,
- depression, grieving,
- assaultive behavior,
- elopement risk,
- self abusive behavior,
- hallucinating behavior,
- delusional behavior,
- withdrawn behavior,
- panic state,
- catatonic state,

5. **Selected nursing diagnoses.** In this case, do not randomly develop protocols for an issue just because it is a nursing diagnosis. Instead, carefully select a half dozen or so issues that are commonly encountered in your patient population and that lend themselves to independent protocol development.

   Essential nursing diagnosis requiring nursing protocols include:

   - alteration in comfort level (chest pain, chronic pain management, or terminal pain management);
   - alteration in mobility (immobility);
   - alteration in level of consciousness (coma);
   - lack of knowledge for self care (any teaching need such as well baby, diabetic instruction, post MI, colostomy care);
   - alteration in nutritional/elimination status (nausea, vomiting, diarrhea, constipation, flatus, anorexia, incontinence);
   - alteration in skin integrity.

These categories are not mutually exclusive nor are they meant to be rigidly interpreted. They simply reflect the extensive range of protocols. In many nursing systems these issues are not addressed at all or are marginally defined in a procedure. Yet much sophisticated nursing care and time revolves around these patient care problems. Think about each category and how it relates to your unit and patient population. You can probably even define additional topics. Remember, however, to control the total number of nursing protocols, first, combine like issues into sections of a single protocol. An example of this is IV Care, where one protocol should comprehensively outline the ongoing management of both peripheral and central lines. Another example is "GI Intubation" where one protocol addresses the care of patients with nasal and/or visceral tubes. Second, separate protocols in generic and unit specific. Most acute nursing systems require approximately 36 generic protocols. While this list may certainly vary from system to system, it provides a good starting point. Expand the list over time as new issues requiring protocols become obvious. The generic protocols are important because they are essential for the medical-surgical areas. They can be used alone or incorporated into standards of care. Also, the speciality areas as MCH or Critical Care will use them. Then, of course, all the specialty areas will develop additional "Unit Specific" protocols to meet the needs of patients in those areas. Table 9-1 lists the 36 topics most often requiring generic protocols.

TABLE 9-1

**Topics Commonly Requiring Generic Protocols**

1. IV Therapy (Central and Peripheral management).
2. Total Parenteral Nutrition (TPN).
3. Tube Feeding.
4. Lipid Infusion.
5. GU Intubation (Indwelling and external urinary device management).
6. GI Intubation (Nasal and visceral tube management).
7. Immobility.
8. Coma.
9. Physiologic Monitoring/Comfort/Hygiene.
10. Hypoglycemia Management.
11. Hypovolemic Shock Management.
12. Seizure Management.
13. Pre-op Care.
14. Post-op Management (including basic pain and wound care).
15. Pre-op Teaching.
16. Colostomy Teaching.
17. Blood Management.
18. Anticoagulant.

19. Insulin Infusion.
20. Anticonvulsant.
21. Artificial Airway (including oral, nasal, trach care).
22. Complicated Wound Management.
23. Alteration in Skin Integrity.
24. Alteration in Nutrition/Elimination Status.
25. Diabetic Teaching.
26. Hypothermia.
27. Oxygen Therapy.
28. Special Beds.
29. Long Term Venous Access Management.
30. Chest Tubes.
31. Restraint.
32. Depression/Grieving.
33. Ostomy Care.
34. Chest pain.
35. Chronic pain.
36. Terminal pain.

Figure 9-2 is a tool that will assist you to identify issues on your own unit. Use it for a week or so when you make rounds and fill in topics that you observe in each category. Get the charge nurses and team members to help. Your list will grow rapidly.

**Protol 1**

*ISSUES FOR PROTOCOL DEVELOPMENT*
(Brainstorming List)

| INVASIVE LINES | NON-INVASIVE EQUIPMENT | THERAPUETIC/ PROPHYLACTIC DIAGNOSTIC MEASURES | PHYSIOLOGIC/ PSYCHOLOGIC STATES | NURSING DIAGNOSIS |
|---|---|---|---|---|
| | | | | |
| | | | | |
| | | | | |
| | | | | |
| | | | | |
| | | | | |
| | | | | |

## Levels of Protocol

Protocols may be classified as dependent, independent, or interdependent. **Dependent Protocols** consist of responsibilities delegated by the medical staff to nursing. These include standing, preprinted, and routine orders. Of course, dependent protocols have become commonplace in critical care units and are gaining acceptance in other areas, such as labor and delivery and psychiatry. Cardiac care units, for example, usually have some established routine delegated to the nursing staff in the event of life-threatening arrhythmias. Emergency drug and treatment orders, such as giving lidocaine for premature ventricular contractions or atropine for bradycardia, fit the definition of a dependent protocol precisely—they direct the nurse in managing a specific patient problem.

Another example of a dependent protocol might be "Hypoglycemia Protocol." While it contains some basic nursing assessment to determine the presence of an insulin reaction as opposed to neurological or cardiopulmonary collapse, the critical intervention is **dependent** as it directs the nurse to actually treat the condition. Study this example in the Protocol section of the Sample Unit Standards Manual and pick out the issues that make it dependent. Generally, two conditions define dependent nursing function. First, the nursing actions involve diagnostic testing, such as ordering lab tests (electrolytes, blood gases) or x-rays (chest film or abdominal flatplate). Second, nursing actions involve medically therapeutic measures using electricity (cardioversion or defibrillation) or pharmacology (ASA, antacids, laxatives, lidocaine, atropine, epinephrine). Identifying dependent protocols is critical because a physican's order must be on the chart before a nurse can carry out the protocol. Obviously, the best time to obtain the order is when the patient is admitted. As the nurse completes her initial admission assessment and reviews the patient's physical condition and identifies initial or potential management problems, she will determine which protocols apply. She can then discuss the use of necessary dependent protocols with the physician and receive a physician's order to carry out the protocol. This acknowledges that when nurses carry out dependent care, they are in the medical practice domain where legal issues require close nurse-physician collaboration and physician sanction of dependent actions.

**Independent Protocols** reflect autonomous nursing functions that require only a nursing order to implement. Examples of titles that are usually independent protocols are "Immobility Protocol," "Chest Tube Protocol," and "Hyperalimentation Protocol."

**Interdependent Protocols** outline management issues that contain both dependent and independent nursing activities. These mixed protocols are often some of the most common that your system might include. As patient acuity increases and nurses seek to expand their roles, combined nursing-medical interventions become more commonplace. Interdependent Protocols require a physician's order prior to implementation, not because of the independent functions, but due to the delegated medical functions. These latter directives are charged to the patient's hospital bill—dietary consult, overhead trapeze, elastic stockings, and so forth. Without a doctor's order, either direct or implied, insurance companies might not pay for these items. Also from a legal standpoint, one could argue that the nurse is functioning out of her jurisdiction. An example of an interdependent protocol is the "Respiratory Protocol" found in the Protocol section in the Unit Standards Manual. Most of the content is strictly autonomous nursing function. However, the dependent issues requiring a physician's order for the protocol include the drawing of blood gases and the ordering of chest x-rays and sputum cultures. If the physician who places the patient on the ventilator wants nursing to pursue these diagnostics measures, then he orders the entire protocol. If he prefers to control these care elements himself, he may so order. In this case, the nursing staff would carry out the independent nursing care only. When writing and using interdependent protocols, it is helpful to place an asterisk next to the dependent functions. This assists the staff in clearly identifying the measures which must be authorized by the patient's physician prior to implementation.

To illustrate the difference between independent and interdependent protocols, consider the following situation. You are taking care of Mr. Jones, who was admitted 12 hours earlier with upper GI bleeding. So far he's shown no sign of bleeding; his hematocrit has been low but stable. But now, when you enter his room to give him his antacid, you find him vomiting bright red blood. His general appearance reflects hypovolemic shock. Managing the patient in shock requires a protocol. But what type of protocol? Independent or interdependent?

In this situation, an independent Shock Protocol would direct you to stay with the patient and to assess his vital signs, airway, and level of consciousness every 3 to 5 minutes. It would also tell you to assess tissue perfusion, position the patient flat, provide pain relief through comfort measures, obtain equipment for resuscitation (such as an IV cutdown tray and crash cart), and place a call to the doctor immediately.

An interdependent Shock Protocol would direct you to carry out the above measure but would include additional dependent interventions such as positioning the patient in the Trendelenberg position, or if respiratory distress develops, with his legs elevated 30 degrees. Other dependent actions might include starting oxygen at 4 liters/minute by cannula; inserting a large-bore (18-gauge) needle in the patient's arm and starting an infusion of 1 liter or normal saline at 250cc/hr; passing a nasogastric tube and beginning saline iced lavage. Interdependent protocols require open communication and negotiation between nurses and doctors to identify clearly the extended role of the nursing staff.

If your system chooses to write and use the Interdependent Shock Protocol, the admitting RN would have to consider that any patient admitted for GI bleeding could hemorrhage and thus might require the shock protocol. The nurse would then raise the possibility with the attending physician, requesting an order for it. If the doctor agrees, the nurse places the verbal order on the doctor's order sheet. All staff now have the permission they require to follow through. If however, the physician chooses not to approve the Interdependent Shock Protocol, staff would be limited to the independent nursing functions. They would not be able to proceed with starting the IV, oxygen, or iced lavage without first calling the physician.

## Points to Consider Before Writing Protocols

**Importance of Levels.** Levels of protocols allow nurses to maintain control over nursing functions. Some hospitals will prefer more conservative independent protocols that strictly limit nursing function; others will encourage more aggressive extended nursing actions, defined by interdependent protocols. Collaborating on content allows nurses to negotiate for what they feel the nursing staff can and should be doing. When this is established in writing, everyone is clear on the extent and limitations of nursing responsibilities. Nurses save time and avoid the frustration of wondering whether they should or should not take certain actions. No longer would nurses have to feel guilty about what they should have done, nor would they have to fear what a doctor might say if they respond to a situation according to protocol. In addition, the interdependent protocol allows the medical staff the decision making freedom they usually demand in controlling what will be done to their patients. Finally, levels of protocols avoid two extremes—nurses not extending themselves into challenging patient care areas (underfunctioning), and nurses overstepping responsibilities and performing unapproved medical actions (overfunctioning).

Several factors will influence the level of the protocol you write. The direction given by your State Nurse Practice Act, for example, must be considered as well as precedents set by community standards of nursing functions. The size and location of your facility is another consideration; small hospitals in rural areas without resident house staff are more likely to require nurses to act aggressively. The sophistication of your nursing staff comes into play. Nursing knowledge and skill levels obviously influence how much responsibility doctors are willing to delegate to nurses. The educational resources available to teach the nursing staff how to deal with complex dependent functions must also be considered. The most important consideration in labeling your protocol as dependent, independent, or interdependent, is obviously *content*. Almost all protocols can be written as independent. This is always the safest way to start! The question then is whether you want to extend the nursing role into the medical domain of dependent functioning of diagnostic and medical therapeutic intervention. This is an important consideration in all nursing care protocols but is especially important in developing emergency response protocols such as shock or seizures.

**Validating Competency.** The more sophisticated and extensive the nursing role within a protocol, the more imperative is documenting staff development to ensure competency. This is true not only in the beginning when the protocol is first implemented, but also over time where infrequent exposure to certain critical situations could compromise both the patient and the nurse. Whenever controversial tasks or responsibilities are accepted with dependent or interdependent protocols, the list of competencies to be validated annually grows. This validation can take place via written examination or simulated situations where staff can be observed and evaluated in terms of their ability to respond with both knowedge and skill demanded by the dependent or interdependent protocol. Lists of nurses proven competent in these demanding areas should be maintained as part of the unit's quality assurance program and then updated yearly.

**Protocols and the Medical Record.** A major consideration is whether protocols should be made a permanent part of the patient's record. Dependent protocols must be part of the record to legally protect the nursing staff and substantiate their use of controversial acts such as defibrillation, pushing IV medication, and intubation. The easiest way to do this is to imprint the dependent protocols onto a physician's order sheet which can then be used for written or verbal orders, the latter being signed within the required 24 hour period. The permanent addition of independent and interdependent protocols is less well defined. Nonetheless, they should be retained in the medical record for five reasons.

First, they define what care the patient required and help justify hospitalization and use of special nursing units. Because discontinuation of protocols and decreasing acuity usually coincide, discharge planning improves as it becomes obvious that the patient no longer requires hospitalization.

Second, when used as a basis for charting, they serve to document nursing care the patient received. Charting by protocol can save valuable nursing time and reduce volume while actually improving the content of notes.

Third, the protocols in the chart can assist third party payors to substantiate nursing costs for time, equipment, supplies, frequency of required interventions, and so forth. By working with insurance companies and other reimbursement agencies to accept documentation by protocols instead of "line item" documentation (where each and every nursing intervention must be separately written in the record), hospitals can ensure the record accurately reflects what was done for the patient. Reimbursement revenues can then be protected or even increased.

Fourth, to work hard at defining our nursing practice and not see it preserved hurts morale.

Finally, the protocols can be used as a basis for retrospective and concurrent quality assurance activities. Data gathering will be easier because the charting will be more complete. Protocols in the record will allow observers to differentiate between documentation difficulties and actual care deficiencies.

To facilitate using protocols and adding to the patient's record, leave space on the protocol for the patient's addressograph. Also create an accountability section at the top indicating the date, time and signature of the RN initiating the protocol. Follow this section with the date, time, and signature of the RN discontinuing the protocol.


| INITIATED | DISCONTINUED |
|-----------|--------------|
| Date _____ | Date _____ |
| Time_____ | Time _____ |
| RN _____ | RN _____ |


While the rationale for maintaining protocols as a permanent part of the patient's record is strong, the Medical Records Department or Committee may still object because of the additional paper volume in the chart. In time, paper records will convert to computerization and then such problems will disappear.

Meanwhile, recognize that you can still write and use your protocols even if they aren't permanent parts of the record. The protocols have been approved legitimately and are a part of your system. They are part of committee minutes and manuals and may be retained in a file in the medical records department. So don't be discouraged if you don't win this small battle—you can still win the war! Use your protocols and try to influence the system later.

### Writing Protocols

In writing protocols, be concise, preferably no more than one page front and back. Go to a second page when the issue is a complex one requiring extensive nursing measures. Resist the temptation to put textbook rationale into the content; protocols should be limited to specific directives for essential nursing actions. Strive to combine brevity and sophistication! Incorporate the expertise of physicians, clinical specialists, senior nursing staff, nursing faculty, and nurse researchers. Consult the latest literature to ensure current content.

When you are writing content, direct nursing actions at both routine and emergency interventions. Always ask yourself "What is the worst thing that could happen to the patient in this situation?" and then address it. The nurse caring for this issue should never be left without direction, should the unthinkable happen! For example, the "Chest Tube Protocol" addresses emergency actions for overflow of drainage systems, accidental dislodgement or disconnection of the tube, excessive air leak, and a tension pneumothorax.

Above all, you want to be as specific as possible in writing protocols. Avoid vague directions or generalizations, such as "Monitor hydration status." Instead, be specific.

Assess hydration status by:

- recording intake and output q̄ 8 hours.
- reporting intake less than 1000 cc/24 hours and reporting urine output less than 1200 cc/24 hours.
- assessing specific gravity of urine each shift and reporting concentration in excess of 1.015.
- noting condition of mucous membranes and skin turgor q̄AM.
- weighing the patient q̄AM.
- assessing for dependent edema in legs and sacrum q̄AM prior to moving patient out of bed.

Also avoid listing information. Instead, turn all relevant information into specific nursing directions. For example, if you were writing a protocol on nitroglycerin, avoid saying "NTG infusion can produce hypotension, headache, and bradycardia." Specific nursing assessment regarding frequency and nursing response would be much more sophisticated and valuable to the staff.

For example:

| Care during infusion | 19. Reassess q̄ 15-minutes as above until positive response obtained; add the following perimeters: |
|---|---|

- perform chest ausculation q̄ 15 minutes if congestion present.
- provide positive feedback about treatment and response.
- stay with patient if he is anxious.
- continue to review rhythm, validating changes with strips in NPR.

Titration    20. Titrate medication to patient response, i.e. clearing chest, decreased SOB, decreased HR, and reduced angina. Recognize there is not set optimum dose—dose/patient response is variable and is a clinical judgment.

Poor Response    21. If no response is seen at 20 mcg/minute, ↑10mcg/minute q̄ 3-5 minutes; *do not exceed* this dose unless directed by physician.

22. If patient is still not responding, inform physician and discuss concommitant use of narcotics or alternate therapy.

Complications    23. Use assessment intervals to validate presence/absence of complications:

*Hypotension (systolic <90 or >30 mm drop in systolic)*

- place patient flat; avoid trendelenburg.
- decrease infusion rate to last level.
- stay with patient and continue decreasing rate to progressive levels until BP stabilizes.
- stop infusion and notify physician if hypotension severe.

*Headache*

- give Tylenol X2 PO (unless NPO/nausea present).
- titrate dose down if severe.
- reduce stimuli; keep bed at 30°.
- notify physician if intolerable, (may have to D/C drip).

*Bradycardia*

- if HR drops but remains >50 without symptoms, observe only.
- if sudden drop or HR <50 creates hypotension, dizziness, or AV dissociation, place flat, administer 0.5 mg atropine IV, and notify physician. Titrate NTG down slowly.

If doctors dispute what you have defined as dependent functions, then adopt a strictly independent focus. In other words, address the controversial issue by focusing on indisputable nursing responsibilities—the nursing process and collaborating with the medical staff. For example, in developing a protocol for caring for patients after cardioversion, the statement, "Use 1% hydrocortisone cream on paddle sites b.i.d. × 3 days," "might be rejected by the medical staff. In that case, a statement to this effect could be substituted: "Assess chest skin for itching, redness and other signs of irritation. If signs are present, discuss the use of a mild steroid topical ointment on affected area with the doctor." Note how this revision converts the proposed dependent action to a strictly independent nursing function with emphasis on nursing assessment and collaboration.

Next, follow a uniform style in writing protocols so they all look and sound consistent. Protocols can be divided into eight components:

| | |
|---|---|
| *TITLE:* | Be as specific as possible, using the word *protocol* to differentiate from other process formats. |
| *PURPOSE:* | Always direct this comment at the care and management of a particular patient problem, situation, or issue. Limit to one sentence. |
| *LEVEL:* | Indicate by using dependent, independent, or interdependent. A brief explanation might be helpful to the staff such as: "Dependent (requires MD order prior to implementation)" or "Interdependent (requires MD order for asterisked dependent functions only.)" |
| *SUPPORTIVE DATA:* | Identify essential information needed to carry out the protocol. Add this only when the issue is new and staff lack experience in the area. Keep it short. Strive to use this component on selected protocols only. |
| *CONTENT STATEMENTS:* | Write the care directives to the *key words* placed to the left. This groups similar interventions, speeds the writing process, and aids the staff in locating specific items. Attempt to address care in a logical or consequential manner. Use a new key word each time you change content topics. |
| *APPROVAL/REVIEW/REVISION:* | Complete information as indicated. |

| | |
|---|---|
| *REFERENCES:* | Limit to one or two. These may include textbooks, journals, or resource persons. |
| *DISTRIBUTION:* | Identify whether the protocol is generic for the department of nursing or specific for certain units. List units where protocol is applicable. |

When writing your key words to brainstorm and organize your content, consider such areas as:

- assessment,
- site checks,
- emergency management,
- tube care,
- infection concerns,
- pain control,
- bedside supplies,
- documentation,
- wound care,
- complications,
- hydration,
- safety concerns,
- reportable concerns,
- electrical precautions,
- patient position.

Finally, as with procedures, it is helpful for staff to use a drafting style when developing protocols. By following the above format, consistency and thoroughness are assured. Remember to include the drafter's name, draft number and date for documentation.

Four examples of protocols using the recommended style are found in the Sample Unit Standards Manual. The first one, "Chest Tube Protocol" is an example of an independent protocol. The second, "Hypoglycemia Protocol" illustrates a totally dependent protocol requiring a doctor's order at admission allowing the staff to implement it. The third, "Respiratory Protocol" is an interdependent protocol with mixed actions, still requiring a physician's order for the dependent functions.

### Writing Teaching Protocols.

Teaching protocols directed at nursing measures to correct patient and family knowledge deficits require special consideration. An additional component should be added to the eight already discussed—outcome standards. Obviously, since patient education can only be evaluated by the patient's response, goals for teaching (or outcome standards) must be written. These are the **only** protocols which require outcome standards. Also, the protocol should serve a dual purpose: to define **what, when,** and **how** some particular aspect of patient education will take place and **document** that it was done and how the patient responded. This combination teaching protocol and teaching record tells the staff member exactly what the patient has been told and where to begin the next teaching session. This is extremely important when busy staff may have only 5 or 10 minutes to engage in patient education activities.

An example of a teaching protocol for "New Colostomy Patients" demonstrates outcome standards by which to evaluate the teaching. It also shows the use of columns to define the protocol teaching steps while simultaneously documenting the events. This would alert all staff caring for a specific patient as to what teaching had been done, what remains to be taught, and the patient's response. There is additional space for more nursing documentation if needed as well as space to enter the date and signature that specified teaching outcomes have been met. This, of course, would need to remain a permanent part of the medical record.

### Using Protocols.

Once protocols have been written and approved, the nursing manager can use them in different ways:

- To orient new staff members to their responsibilities in specific situations.

Using protocols for orientation promotes safe, effective and appropriate patient care. It also prevents new staff members from assuming that what they did in their previous place of employment is appropriate on your unit.

- To upgrade the role of the RN in patient care.

If you want patient care on your unit to be more sophisticated, you can define these higher levels of functioning in protocols, educate your staff to them, and then evaluate staff members according to this higher level of practice. Defining nursing functions in written protocols reduces anxiety among staff members in new situations by giving them specific directions. If your staff had to learn hemodynamic pressure monitoring, for example, you would not only have to teach them about the equipment and techniques of assisting the physician, but you would also want to define ongoing patient care management. Written protocols for dealing with routine and emergency situations help you direct your staff properly and protect your patients from harm.

- *To promote staff development.*

Protocols can be used to plan continuing education sessions for new or complex nursing activities and to update staff members on infrequent aspects of care. They can serve as a basis for testing your staff's knowledge of required nursing responses in specific situations, thus validating staff competency in high risk care.

- *To facilitate quality assurance.*

Periodically staff compliance to existing protocols needs to be evaluated. Protocols can facilitate the activity, by serving as legitimate sources of review criteria, allowing staff performance and patient care to be appraised in a consistent and accurate manner.

### Operationalizing Protocols.

One of the most critical decisions to be made concerning protocols is how the nursing staff will use them. Of course, you want to organize your protocols in your Unit Standards Manual, but this is not enough. You want the protocols to be more accessible—as close to the nurse, patient, and care planning system as possible. The objective is to set up a mechanism where the staff will use the protocols at the patient's bedside. One option is to create and maintain a file cabinet on each nursing unit. A two drawer cabinet is best, using the top drawer for your protocols and the bottom for your standards of care, next on our discussion agenda. The protocol drawer would be organized alphabetically and contain approximately one dozen copies of each protocol applicable to your unit. For example, "C" would contain protocols on chest tubes, central lines, cardioversion, cast care, and so forth. A unit clerk would be assigned to maintain the cabinet.

After determining that a certain protocol should be followed for a particular patient, the nurse would simply go to the file, select the required protocol(s) and individualize them. Individualization means validating that the protocol is appropriate for the patient and the situation. Defining mechanisms to individualize the protocol is essential to prevent "rubber stamping," or indiscriminately using the protocols failing to make sure they fit the situation. In order to combat the mistaken notion that individualization means significant rewriting, the specific measures for individualization must be clearly defined. The major emphasis is on "thinking and matching the content" to the patient, not writing a lot of content.

### Mechanisms for Individualization of Protocols

- addressograph the protocol with the patient's name, indicating the protocol is part of the patient's care.
- enter the date, time, and signature when the protocol is initiated and discontinued, making the staff accountable for following the content.
- read the protocol carefully and add, delete, or modify it as needed.

Let's look at an example of individualization of a protocol. You are taking care of an elderly woman who is receiving intravenous therapy for maintenance fluid and antibotic administration. Therefore you would be following the "IV Therapy Protocol," specifically the section on peripheral IV's as opposed to central lines. Suppose the protocol directs the staff to rotate the IV site every 72 hours in order to prevent phlebitis. You know that it required several insertion attempts before being successful with this current line and that the doctor would probably have to resort to a central line or cutdown if this line is lost. The protocol also directs you to use an iodine preparation in daily site care and your patient is allergic to this substance. Then it would be prudent for you to modify the protocol in both areas by writing the specific alterations directly on the protocol itself so all staff would be aware of the change in this patient's IV care. You would direct your coworkers to maintain the present site until obvious signs of inflammation or infiltration occurred, while carrying out rigid daily care and inspection. You would also change the iodine routine to an alternate regimen such as cleansing with alcohol only.

This example illustrates a very important point. Protocols can save nursing time and energy while improving care, if they are used properly. Written individualization is essential to prevent abuse. Both managers and staff must understand that once a protocol is selected and put into practice, it must be followed as it is written or professionally modified in writing. This means that each professional practitioner providing care has both the prerogative and obligation to alter a protocol as long as the mechanisms are defined and followed.

The protocol would then be placed into the patient's Kardex, chart, patient care management binder, or bedside clipboard. Notation in record would indicate any changes in the protocol that were made. It would stay there as long as it applies to the patient's care, providing direction and a basis for documentation and evaluation. Depending on patient acuity, some patients would have only one or two protocols in effect at any point in time, while sicker patients might have four or five protocols. However, since acuity changes quickly on most patients and lengths of stay in acute facilities are so short, many protocols would not be in effect for more than a couple of days. Head nurses, supervisors or charge nurses can assess patients' needs during rounds and validate that these protocols are indeed in effect and being evaluated and documented. Thus using protocols in this manner provides a built in accountability system for supervision and QA. In addition, of course, it removes assumption that all staff operate in the same manner. It also prevents staff from having to spend valuable time writing down repetitive care issues.

When the protocol is no longer applicable, it would be removed from the bedside and placed behind the nursing progress records where it would remain a permanent part of the chart. Of course, if that cannot be negotiated with the Medical Records Department, the protocol would be discarded.

If your system is progressive in its computerization, then your nursing station or bedside computer can take the place of the "manual file cabinet." The computer would be programmed with the protocols, which could be called up, individualized on the screen, and then printed for use.

### Mechanisms for Professional Modification of Protocols

All modifications:

- are in writing on the protocol including date and signature of responsible person.
- include explanation of and rationale for the change in the nursing progress notes so staff will understand the nature and reason for the change.
- are evaluated for effectiveness in the nursing progress notes on a shift basis.

Supervisory staff should monitor the frequency and nature of professional modifications made by the staff. If few are made, this could indicate inadequate individualization; if certain areas are consistently changed by the staff, consideration should be given to permanently revising the content through appropriate channels.

Finally, in order to direct the staff in the successful use of protocols at the bedside, directives guiding individualization and professional modification must be captured in written "Guidelines for Use of Protocols and Standards of Care". These will be further discussed in the next chapter.

We've seen then how procedures provide step-by-step instructions for performing nursing tasks, while protocols provide sophisticated and specific direction for managing five areas of patient problems or issues. Together they form a large portion of your process standards. There are two more formats to round out the process standards—guidelines and standards of care.

# Chapter 10:  Guidelines and Standards of Care

## GUIDELINES

Guidelines tell you how to use a nursing tool properly. Nursing tools include data bases, flow sheets, vital signs records, intake and output sheets, medications sheets, transfer forms, nursing progress records, narcotics records, assignment worksheets, and so forth. Their purpose is to facilitate effective documentation, record-keeping, and communication. This fifth format of Process Standards can help orient your new staff members to their documentation responsibilities and provide the basis for inservicing new nursing chart forms. Guidelines can also be the source of audit criteria for evaluating the accuracy and sophistication of charting as a part of your unit's quality assurance activities. Essentially, guidelines should exist for all nursing department and unit communications and documentation forms. Guidelines should be maintained in your Unit Standards Manual to serve as a constant reference for your staff in directing good documentation.

The term **guideline** is often used loosely in nursing to mean a "suggestion". The Marker Model rejects the notion that any standard is merely a suggestion. Guidelines are serious standards, addressing the business of record keeping. To refer to directions for using forms as procedures is inappropriate. Legal and professional requirements for documentation should not be reduced to a technical task. Rather, the use of forms and tools is a complex responsibility and must be defined by a sophisticated process format. Thus, to insert an indwelling bladder catheter and measure the eight hour urinary volume is a procedure; however, we define how the "Intake and Output Record" will be completed to reflect the patient's hydration and elimination status in guidelines. To administer heparin or coumadin is a procedure, but guidelines define the use of the "Anticoagulant Flowsheet" to record and coordinate drug therapy, timing, and patient response.

### Writing Guidelines

The best persons to write guidelines are the staff because they do the charting and they know the details—and details are the secret to a good set of guidelines. In our last discussion on procedures and protocols, we stressed brevity. Length was an important issue in procedure development because of their volume and a critical issue in protocol writing because the staff uses protocols to provide care at the bedside. However, length is not an issue in guidelines development—in fact effective guidelines may be very extensive in order to provide the necessary direction in filling out nursing forms.

Your guidelines should include ten components.

| | |
|---|---|
| *TITLE:* | Use the word "Guidelines" in the title to differentiate from other process formats. |
| *PURPOSE:* | The purpose is always to direct the nurse in accurate documentation. |
| *NATURE:* | Specify whether the form is a permanent or temporary worksheet. If permanent, provide details about addressographing, use and color of ink, use of both sides of paper. |
| *DEFINITIONS:* | Explain new or unusual terms. If none, omit this section. |
| *PATIENT POPULATION:* | Identify for which patients the form is to be used and under which circumstances. Be specific. |
| *RESPONSIBLE PERSONS:* | Indicate who is responsible for initiating the tool—nurse or unit secretary—and who completes the form. This pinpoints accountability when multiple persons are involved. |
| *CHART PLACEMENT:* | Specify where the form goes and who should put it there. |
| *DETAILED INSTRUCTIONS:* | Divide the form into sections and fill out each section labeling it "example." Cut the sections into pieces. Now write a detailed explanation of how to fill in each section, pasting each completed section immediately after the set of directions. Two copies of the entire form should be attached, one blank and one complete. |
| *APPROVAL/REVIEW/REVISION:* | Complete dates and mechanisms. |

*DISTRIBUTION:* Specify whether form is generic to department of nursing or unit specific and where it may be found.

If you incorporate each of these components, you will have a set of guidelines that defines the form, specifies how it is to be used, and tells the nurse how to complete it. Your content tells her what to do, your examples show her how it's supposed to look. The easiest mistake to make in writing guidelines is not being specific enough. The test of a good set of guidelines is whether a nurse who has never seen the form before can read the guidelines and complete the form correctly.

As with the past two process formats, drafting expedites writing guidelines while teaching staff how to do them better in the future. "Guidelines for Completing the Anticoagulant Flowsheet," found under Process Standards in the Sample Unit Standards Manual, illustrates a useful level of detail and the proper use of instructional directions.

## STANDARDS OF CARE

Standards of Care define the care for groups of patients about whom generalizations and predictions can be made. These are the most sophisticated process standards you will write. They are different from any process format yet discussed. Performance standards are directed at defining expectations of the nursing staff, extending job descriptions beyond their narrow range. Procedures address nursing tasks; protocols define nursing management of broad issues or problems in five areas, and Standards of Care are directed at **patient population groups**. A population group is a collection of patients who have common nursing care needs directly or indirectly related to a specific pathology entity. A patient population group can be labeled according to:

- admitting diagnosis,
- discharge diagnosis,
- medical diagnosis,
- diagnosis related group (DRG).

If you ask your Medical Records Department to give you a list of the top dozen DRGs admitted to your unit last year, you would have the starting place for patient populations that require Standards of Care for your area. Begin with the top four and proceed until you have completed the dozen. You can then turn your attention to the least common patients on your unit. This approach is effective because it defines care for patients who consume the majority of your hours of nursing care and equipment/supply budget, and frees the staff from excess writing. It also reduces stress and chance of error when staff care for patients they rarely see. Over time you can develop a sufficient number of standards of care to bring the two extremes together! You are working toward a point where the majority of patients admitted to your area will have a preprinted standard of care ready and waiting to be pulled and individualized. This meets both our professional responsibilities for care planning and maximizes use of staff time. Examples of patient populations requiring standards of care might be Congestive Heart Failure, Hypertension, Laminectomy,

Gastritis, Barbiturate Overdose, Total Hip Replacement, and Diabetes Mellitus.

Because standards of care demand sophisticated use of nursing process and deal with groups of patients, they are at the top of the process standards and are the last to be developed. They incorporate all other process standards.

Many nursing systems have tried to develop standard care plans but have had difficulty using them because they have been repetitive, over long, and not individualized or consistently used by the nursing staff. In order to be successful, standards of care must meet certain requirements. They must:

1. Be limited to four sides (two pages front and back).
2. Be integrated with existing protocols to prevent unnecessary duplication of content.
3. Have their use clearly defined in written guidelines.
4. Be actively supervised by both staff and nursing management to reward compliance and nip non-compliance in the bud.
5. Become part of the unit's quality assurance program to monitor effectiveness and insure continued compliance and accountability on the part of the staff.

Standards of care are the last stage of process standards development so that all other Process pieces are in place to support that standard of care. Generally speaking, your system should have in place or be developing approximately thirty generic protocols before beginning to write standards of care. Your standards of care will go smoother and faster and give you a mechanism to control length when you have accumulated well written protocols on common issues and problems your patients and staff face daily.

### Style and Characteristics.

You can use one of the two styles to write standards of care: the **Standard Care Plan** (SCP) and the **Standard Care Statement** (SCS). These two styles give you flexibility in adjusting standards of care to your staff's level of care planning and to your type of unit. You can choose one style over the other or mix them, using one style for some groups of patients and another style on other groups of patients.

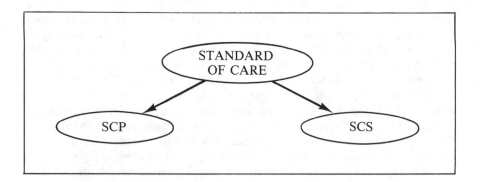

Certain characteristics, however, must apply to any style of standard of care you select. Specifically, all standards of care must:

- **Be directed at diagnostic categories of patients only, not issues within that patient population, and be integrated with existing protocols.**

  For example, provide a standard of care for the patient with CVA, Spinal Cord Injury, and Thrombophlebitis but a "Protocol for Immobility." Since all three patient populations are permanently or temporarily immobile, "impaired physical mobility" would be listed as one priority nursing problem in the standard of care for each patient population. The intervention would direct you to "follow the Immobility Protocol," but would not repeat the nursing care listed in that protocol. The standard of care would then define other pertinent nursing problems/diagnoses and spell out interventions for which no protocol has been written.

  Again, provide a standard of care for the Gastrectomy Patient, the Total Hip Replacement Patient, and the Carotid Endarterectomy Patient but a "Protocol for Post-Operative Management." All three patient populations are post-op and thus all three Standards of Care would state as a nursing diagnosis, "altered physiologic state related to post-op condition" and tell you to "adhere to the Post-Op Protocol," but would not repeat the specific protocol directives. The standards of care would, however, go on to spell out other problems and care required within each diagnostic category.

- **Be limited to two pages each (front and back).**

  This becomes critical because too much paper undermines the use of the standards of care. Control length by:

  1. limiting the nursing diagnoses dealt with in each patient population to about 6;
  2. eliminating all rationale content and making nursing intervention specific, essential, and concise; and
  3. integrating existing protocols into nursing interventions as opposed to repeating content as demonstrated by the above examples.

- **Be operationalized at the bedside for use by all staff on each shift.**

- **Contain Outcome Standards by which to evaluate results of care.**

- **Be capable of being individualized and updated by the nursing staff.**

A standard care plan (SCP) describes the essential physiological, psychological, and cognitive care to be given to a group of patients. This formal, sophisticated tool is organized into columns and follows the form sequence of the nursing process. SCPs specify key nursing diagnoses characteristic of a DRG (pathologic entity). For each nursing diagnosis, a nursing goal or patient outcome is stated along with the nursing actions designed to achieve both the nursing and patient outcomes.

A standard care statement (SCS) is a list of interventions describing the care required by a group of patients. It is less formal than an SCP because no columns are used; nursing actions are simply grouped around subject headings. However, the nursing actions should be just as specific, comprehensive, and sophisticated as in an SCP. An SCS is also less formal than an SCP in that specific nursing diagnoses are not used and outcome standards are not written for each entry. Instead, general patient outcomes directed at the patient population as a whole are given. This still allows for outcome reviews to be done.

Many nurses find standard care statements easier to write and choose to develop standard care plans only for their major patient populations. SCSs lend themselves to short stay, rapid turnover areas such as the PAR, Labor and Delivery, OR, and ER. Reserve formal SCPs for bedded units such as ICU, CCU, Medical-Surgical Units, and Psychiatry.

Remember, in selecting your patient populations for standards of care, include the patients you care for the most often to ensure consistency and prevent *routine* from becoming synonomous with *haphazard*. Be sure to develop standards of care for those patient groups that you rarely admit because the staff may lack sophisticated knowledge in these areas due to infrequent exposure. Your list of DRGs may come from the Medical Records Department or your unit log. Once you've decided which patients to work on, you'll have to decide which style to use. As with past process formats, drafting is the quickest way to help the staff give you good results. Finally, examples of an SCP and an SCS are provided under process standards in the Sample Unit Standards Manual to compare these two different styles.

Before you actually start to write standards of care, look carefully at your present nursing care Kardex. In many cases, this is your best drafting form! If your Kardex is to your liking, then use it! Just make several hundred copies of the nursing care plan portion and have the staff draft SCPs directly on them. Then finalize them for typing and print the final SCP on the form. This way the SCPs look just like the regular Kardexes and staff confusion will be non-existent. However, it is essential that your present Kardex contain the following characteristics.

- addressograph location;
- initiate and discontinue sections for the entire SCP;
- mechanisms for identifying nursing diagnoses, outcomes, and nursing interventions;
- mechanisms for activating (starting) and deactivating (stopping) a particular nursing diagnosis;
- mechanisms for evaluating care each 24 hour period and communicating that this has been done.


*Developing Standard Care Plans.*

In developing standard care plans, follow these steps:

1. **Select your patient populations.**

2. **Select the style most appropriate for your unit and needs.** If you choose the SCP, you'll have to determine the number of columns, two, three, or four. The two column approach has limitations, while four columns

require extra work and time to complete. Three columns address all nursing process steps yet facilitate writing. Let's look at each style.

The four column approach is the most extensive layout. It places nursing diagnosis in the initial column and nursing intervention in the last column, with the two middle columns used to address outcome standards, both nursing goals and patient outcomes. Writing both levels of outcome statements requires expertise and commitment. It is ultimately the most sophisticated approach.

| NURSING DIAGNOSIS / PATIENT CARE PROBLEM | NURSING GOAL | PATIENT OUTCOME | NURSING INTERVENTION |
|---|---|---|---|
|  |  |  |  |

The three column approach omits Nursing Goals. Since many nurses don't write nursing goals because they feel they are redundant with patient outcomes, you may elect to address patient outcomes only. This shortens the writing time but still directs the plan and provides the basis for outcome review.

| NURSING DIAGNOSIS / PATIENT CARE PROBLEM | PATIENT OUTCOME | NURSING INTERVENTION |
|---|---|---|
|  |  |  |

The two column approach focuses entirely on nursing diagnosis and nursing interventions, but no care plan is complete without outcome standards. So in this approach, the outcome statements are written at the bottom of each column. Unfortunately, the terms "Short-term Goals" and "Long-term Goals" still appear on some Kardexes. These two phrases offer little direction to the nursing staff. They are very subjective, leaving the nurse to decide for herself just what "short-term" and "long-term" mean. Obviously, they mean something very different in a recovery room setting compared to a medical-surgical unit.

Therefore, they should be eliminated and replaced with the more meaningful terms, nursing goals and patient outcomes. Nursing goals are "staff oriented" and focus on what nursing is trying to accomplish. Patient outcomes are "patient oriented" and are statements of conditions reflecting desired changes in the patient.

| NURSING DIAGNOSIS | | NURSING INTERVENTION |
|---|---|---|
| PATIENT CARE PROBLEMS | | |
| | Nursing Goals | Patient Outcomes |

Regardless of your approach, your standards of care must follow the nursing process by using the first column for "Nursing Diagnosis" and the last column for "Nursing Interventions", connecting the two with "Outcome Standards."

Some Kardexes are inappropriately designed. This occurs in several ways. First, outcome standards are placed last. This often results in staff planning care prior to, or even totally without, specifying what is to be accomplished. This, of course, violates nursing process and means the plan has no direction toward a pre-specified end. Defining outcomes was an afterthought. Second, a column is used to specify "Evaluation." The use of this column is poorly defined and its size invites narrative writing. This is inappropriate because the care plan is the tool used to define care, update, and resolve care, not to express evaluation of effectiveness. Nursing progress records are the proper location for this. Of course, no staff nurse wants to write content twice! Reserve any columns titled "Evaluation" for dates and signatures only, not content. Third, some Kardex formats delineate sections for short term, long term, outcomes, discharge goals, and teaching goals. This is the ultimate in redundancy! Eliminate all issues but "Outcome Standards" as these can be used to achieve all physiologic, psychologic, and cognitive ends for the patient.

3. **Title the SCP.** Make it complete using "Standard of Care" to differentiate it from a protocol and specifying the style of SCP or SCS. Include the DRG addressed. For example, "Standard of Care (SCP) for Patients with CHF" or "Standard of Care (SCS) for Patients with Thrombophlebitis."

4. **Identify 6 Priority Nursing Diagnoses.** While certain patient populations may be so complex that they require a greater number of nursing diagnoses, the majority of your DRGs should be developed within this limit. We must keep emphasizing that the goal is brevity and sophistication. The standards of care must be realistic and achievable within our

shorter hospital stays. Direct the initial four nursing diagnoses at key **physiologic problems**; use the fifth nursing diagnosis to define the priority **psychologic problem**; use the sixth to address the main **cognitive need** of the patient and significant others. Combine several problems under one nursing diagnosis to save time and space. For example, instead of separating alterations in elimination, potential alterations in skin integrity, and potential alterations in ventilatory status, you might relate all these potential problems to "Immobility." Emphasize staff focus on the initial 72 hours of hospitalization or care. Additional patient care concerns that are identified can always be added to the SCP or Kardex as a mechanism of individualization. How you state your nursing diagnoses is up to your system and chosen literature resources. Additionally, you notice that in demonstrating the different column styles of SCP's the initial nursing diagnosis column is dual titled as "Nursing Diagnosis/Patient Care Problem". This is to allow staff to use existing nursing diagnosis language according to their expertise but also allow staff to state other legitimate nursing concerns as "problems." Given the current status of nursing diagnosis, this option seems advisable.

5. **Identify Outcome Standards.** The column approach chosen will determine the extensiveness of your outcome standards: nursing goals and patient outcomes, or patient outcomes only.

6. **Specify Nursing Interventions.** Be specific, using short, precise statements to provide direction for nursing actions. Avoid using vague or superficial statements such as "watch patient for bleeding," unless you specify how to do this. Do not use words such as "PRN" and "if necessary" as these do not define care. Do not leave blanks to be filled in arbitrarily by the staff. These approaches do not represent standards. Write all nursing measures using numbers to list care just as it should be given, giving times, frequencies, and exact actions. Using abbreviations acceptable to your system will also expedite writing. After you have defined the care, number the next two lines and leave them blank, inviting the staff to add or alter care as mechanisms for individualization. Remember that the individualization mechanism will allow staff to modify the standard of care as necessary for any particular patient.

A common error in standard care plan writing is for staff to communicate information instead of directing care. An example would be the statement, "Be aware that CHF causes sodium and fluid retention with exudation into pulmonary and subcutaneous interstitium and low specific gravity." While this is a true reflection of failure pathology, it does not tell the staff what to do. Instead, the nursing intervention should direct the staff to assess for sodium and fluid retention and state how to do so in terms of chest auscultation, daily weights, monitoring of specific gravity, urinary output, and presence of dependent edema. Obviously, in the statement, "watch patient for bleeding," the same message applies: get more specific and sophisticated.

Nursing interventions should contain both independent and dependent functions. As before, if dependent functions are blocked, convert them to independent actions, focusing on nursing process and collaboration with the medical staff. For example, if you were writing an SCP on a patient with thrombophlebitis, ordering anticoagulants is not within the nursing domain. However, the SCP should still address the possibility of pulmonary embolization and direct the nursing staff to discuss the possibility of anticoagulants with the physician. This example brings up the final point in writing interventions. Remember to reduce the amount of writing by integrating existing protocols. Thus one part of the SCP might look like this:

| NURSING DIAGNOSIS | PATIENT OUTCOME | NURSING INTERVENTION |
|---|---|---|
| 4. Potential for altered cardiac status related to possible pulmonary emboli. | The patient will maintain stable cardiac and pulmonary function to promote adequate ventilation and tissue perfusion. | 1. Assess chest sounds q̄ shift for congestion.<br>2. Record rate and character of respirations 2X per shift.<br>3. Report/record SOB, cough, hemoptysis, or respiratory rate > 24 min.<br>4. Instruct patient to save all sputum in bedside container and notify staff of any dyspnea, tachypnea, or hemoptysis.<br>5. Maintain position of Semi-fowlers.<br>6. Discuss with MD the use of anticoagulants; if patient to be anticoagulated, follow "Anticoagulant Protocol." |

7. **Add Approval, Review, and Revision Dates.**

8. **Indicate One or Two Main References.**

9. **Specify Distribution. This indicates where the SCP can be found and which units will be using it.**

*Developing Standard Care Statements.*

The steps in developing standard care statements are similar to those discussed in writing SCPs but with a few differences:

1. **Identify Your Patient Populations.**

2. **Adopt A Style of SCS.** This is less rigid and formal than the SCP but needs its own "appearance and characteristics" for ready staff recognition. Nursing interventions are grouped around subject headings so the care statements will be organized and prioritized. Outcome standards are listed at the top as broad statements of physiologic, pyschologic, and cognitive status to be achieved. To take the place of a sophisticated SCP evaluation mechanism, a simple space for "date met and signature" works. Obviously, a "start" and "stop" column activates and

deactivates nursing care measures. Because SCSs are used primarily in short stay areas on relatively uncomplicated patients, SCSs are usually limited to one page, front and back. Of course, they can also be used on seriously ill diagnostic categories and would be longer.

| Outcome Standard:  Physiologic:  Psychologic:  Cognitive: | | | Date Met/Signature: | | |
|---|---|---|---|---|---|

| Initiated | | Subject Heading | Nursing Intervention | Discontinue | |
| Date | RN | | | Date | RN |
| | | | | | |

3. **Title the SCS.** Make the title complete.

4. **Establish General Outcome Standards.** Instead of writing an outcome for each nursing diagnosis, simply develop three general patient outcome statements at the top of the SCS, relating them to the patient's physiological, psychological, and cognitive status. These will still give a focus to the standard of care and provide for the development of outcome criteria at the time outcome review is done.

5. **Identify Major Subject Headings.** These subject headings are general issues of concern to the nursing staff or anticipated problems common to the DRG, or, if you prefer, they could be stated as nursing diagnoses to give the SCS a more sophisticated level. Generally, however, this list consists of topical headings because some nurses have found dealing with general concerns easier than dealing with specific nursing diagnoses. These headings allow you to organize care statements rather than haphazardly listing care. This approach also allows quick reference to particular aspects of nursing care. Common topical headings would be: assessment, wound/tube care, complications, documentation, patient teaching, reportable conditions to the doctor, psychological support, nutritional or elimination needs, and so forth.

6. **Write Nursing Care Statements.** List and number nursing measures around appropriate headings. Follow the same concept as discussed under SCPs. The definition of nursing care must be just as complete and specific.

7. **Add Approval, Review, and Revision Dates.**

8. **Include References, only one or two.**

9. **Specify Distribution.**

*Resistance to Pre-Written Plans of Care.*

Before we begin this discussion, let's clarify some confusing points of terminology. **Standards of Care** are pre-written plans of care for a group (DRG) of patients. **Individual care plans** start as blank Kardexes and force the nursing staff to write all care plans from "scratch." The term **individualized care plan** means the plan of care has been judged to meet the specific needs of a particular patient. The terms "individual" and "individualized" are commonly confused. Individualized care is what patients require and nurses strive to deliver. Therefore, standards of care are indeed meant to replace individual (from scratch) care plans because individual care plans have not worked in the past and are not working now. Because of the realities of hospital nursing today, individual care plans are not the answer to care planning in the future. What standards of care will accomplish, among other things, is to make the obligation of individualized care planning a reality.

Nurses have struggled with individual care plans for decades and still the "blank Kardex syndrome" persists. The idea of using pre-written standardized care plans is accepted by some and rejected by others. Occasionally, nursing systems reject SCPs because of a bad experience with them in the past. The SCPs, however, are not always the cause of the problem. The "culprit" that leads to their failure may be in the system, if the SCPs are not properly written and their use is not clearly defined and monitored. Standards of care must be seen not only as a means to define what we mean by safe, effective, and appropriate patient care, but also as a tool to help nurses work smarter not harder.

Look at the realities of today's hospital nursing: less staff, sicker patients, and shorter lengths of stay. All combine to make the burden of care planning as it has been traditionally approached even more unrealistic. Add to these problems the fact that many nurses lack the skill to write a concise, relevant, and sophisticated plan of care on any "DRG" to which they are assigned. This leads to the current dilemma of frustrated nurse managers and hasseled staff, both viewing individual care plans as time-consuming, boring (especially writing the same things on the same types of patients day after day), dispensable, superficial in content, impossible to keep current or to use to hold staff members accountable. As long as nurses are expected to write individual care plans from scratch for every patient, the job will continue to be done haphazardly, varying with each nurse's capabilities and doing little to promote quality, continuity, and consistency.

Now consider these advantages to use pre-written standards of care:

- They're more interesting to use because the routine care has already been written, which saves a lot of time and allows the nurse to concentrate on "individualizing" the plan to suit her patient. Sometimes the plan is so applicable to the patient that no modification is necessary at all.

- They can be kept as a permanent part of the patient's record instead of being discarded, which should boost staff morale. They will also be available for future reference if the patient is readmitted.

- Their content is sophisticated because the plan was written by nurses who took their time, took advantage of care experts, such as clinical specialists, faculty members, nurse researchers, and so forth, and consulted the literature. They haven't been dashed off under the stress of everyday nursing responsibilities and 2:45 PM admissions.

- Accountability is not a problem because the care plan has been worked out by a group, not just one nurse. (Consider the natural reluctance to initial Kardex entries for fear of ridicule from coworkers—the old "safety-in-anonymity" routine.)

To illustrate these advantages in action, let's examine a situation:

A 73 year old woman is transferred to a busy medical-surgical unit from the recovery room after undergoing a gastrectomy. She has a Foley catheter, CVP line, gastrectomy tube, and is receiving total parenteral nutrition. She had an MI only six months ago, but the abdominal surgery was too urgent to postpone. This patient has been a diabetic for 30 years and has an above-the-knee amputation, successfully fitted with prosthesis. She is quite active and uses the artificial limb effectively.

The staff nurse assigned to this patient will be hard-pressed to get her admitted, assessed, and comfortable, to take report from the recovery room, to carry out essential physician orders, and to complete the initial postop admission nursing notes and flow sheet activities. She'll be lucky to get all this done while caring for her other patients, administering medications, charting, and giving report on time. Unless this nurse is especially knowledgeable, organized, and experienced, she'll likely be putting in some overtime. Where will this patient's care plan rank on the nurse's list of priorities?

Basically, the nurse has three options in response to the "blank Kardex syndrome":

1. Leave it blank and hope someone on the next shift will fill it out.

2. Write something just to fill up the space. Given the limited time and thought, the content will undoubtedly be superficial. If the nurse in our example knows little about gastrectomy patients, the content will be very general indeed. And what would she write about the TPN? Probably nothing. "Oh well, everyone on the unit knows all that stuff anyway," she might say to herself. Just get the basic issues down like pain, drainage, turn-cough - deep breathe. What about the secondary diagnoses of diabetes and coronary artery disease? Forget it — no time.

3. Or, in less than 10 minutes, the nurse could pull the following standards on file in the unit:

- Standard Care Plan for Gastrectomy Patients,
- TPN Protocol,

- GI Intubation Protocol,
- IV Therapy Protocol

These standards could be addressographed, dated and initialed, and read over quickly for applicability to the patient, then modified as the nurse sees fit. She could affix the SCP and protocols to the patient's Kardex to direct essential care during the first 48 to 72 hours. She could then use the Kardex to address secondary issues such as stump care, urine and blood glucose testing, daily weights, and so forth.

Now, which option sounds most realistic in this situation? It all boils down to staff capabilities, available time, and appropriate use of resources. To expect staff members to deal with routine care in a sophisticated manner and also thoroughly address individualized aspects of care from scratch is simply not realistic.

### Avoiding Pitfalls.

As helpful as standards of care are, four pit falls can undermine their use and lead to problems with accrediting agencies such as JCAH:

1. Failure to integrate the standards of care into the care planning system.

2. Tendency of staff to "rubber stamp" prewritten plans, failing to individualize them to the patient.

3. Failure of the system to define precisely how standards of care and associated protocols will be used.

4. Lack of a consistent monitoring system for accountability.

**Failure to integrate Standards of Care into the care planning system** occurs when the standards of care are placed in a manual on the unit and no provision is made for literally using them as a basis for giving care. This produces a paper system and results in defined care being "out of sight, out of mind." Kardexes are still blank and care is not improved. Prevent this error by creating and using a standard of care and protocol filing system. This can be a manual or computerized. A manual system should be used for a year or so before computer commitment is made. In relation to a manual system of "pulling" standards, remember our two-drawer file cabinet in the nurse's station? The first drawer was labeled protocols; the second drawer should be labeled standards of care. In this second drawer are a dozen copies of each standard of care to be used on your unit, arranged alphabetically according to patient populations group. Each staff member then pulls the appropriate standard of care for her patient as soon as possible after admission to the unit. Protocols are also selected which support the standard of care. After individualization, they are put where they will be *used*—on the Kardex, chart, or bedside clipboard. As with protocols, the standard of care will stay there as long as it applies to the patient, then be discarded or made a permanent part of the patient's record. The same arguments for making the protocols part of the record apply to standards of care. This setup, or something similarly suited to your unit, will make your standards of care and protocols an integral and natural part of your care planning system. You are replacing questionable "writing from scratch" practices with a "professional selection of existing standards" approach. Professional judgment and decision making skills are enhanced.

This facilitates a higher level of functioning by the nursing staff. Careful nursing judgment is required to detemine which standards of care and protocols are best suited to direct the care of a particular patient. More decision making is necessary to specify which standards will be modified and what additional or altered care will make the standards applicable to a patient. Use of nursing process is enhanced because standards of care and protocols can be selected, modified, and maintained only in conjunction with sophisticated patient assessment.

In order to overcome this tendency of staff to **"rubber stamp" pre-written plans failing to individualize them to the patient,** it is essential to spell out exactly what individualization is and how it is to be done. Individualizing a standard of care is not synonymous with rewriting content; while some steps use only the pen or pencil, most use the brain. The essence of individualization requires the RN to initiate the plan, validate that it applies to the patient or modify it so it does, keep it up-to-date, and use it as a basis for evaluating care. The design of the standard of care tool itself can facilitate these activities.

These steps of individualization include:

1. Addressographing the standard of care to mark it for a specific patient.

2. Entering the date the standard of care was put into effect and the signature of the responsible RN to ensure accountability.

3. Activating the nursing diagnoses (or problems) by date and initial as they become relevant.

4. Reading the content for applicability and modifying it as necessary by adding, deleting, or altering nursing measures.

5. Evaluating the ongoing problems daily to determine whether each problem is still active or resolved, modifying care as necessary.

6. Deactivating nursing diagnoses as they are resolved, using date and initials.

7. Entering the date the standard of care is discontinued, usually when the patient is transferred to another unit or discharged home.

The three column example below shows how style can facilitate these steps.

| HOSPITAL<br>DEPARTMENT OF NURSING<br>STANDARD OF CARE (SCP) ON THE PATIENT<br>WITH: *Thrombophlebitis* | | | | INITIATED<br>Date: _____<br>Time: _____<br>RN: _____ | | | DISCONTINUED<br>Date: _____<br>Time: _____<br>RN: _____ | | |
|---|---|---|---|---|---|---|---|---|---|
| INITIATED | | NURSING DIAGNOSIS | PATIENT OUTCOME | EVALUATED | | NURSING | RESOLVED | | |
| Date | Initials | PATIENT CARE PROBLEMS | | Date | Initials | INTERVENTIONS | Date | Initials | |
|  |  |  |  |  |  |  |  |  | |

The example allows each nursing diagnosis to be activated independently based on the nurse's assessment of her patients, and then evaluated each 24 hours. If a nursing diagnosis is initiated on 8/24, then 8/25 is entered in the EVALUATED column. Automatically, the responsible RN re-evaluates the problem on 8/25. Either the problem is resolved on that date or it is ongoing. If resolved, then 8/25 is entered in the RESOLVED column. If ongoing, then 8/25 is changed to 8/26 and re-evaluation takes place again on 8/26 and so forth until final resolution occurs. The Evaluation column can be maintained in pencil and completed in pen or maintained in pen and scratched through with a new date. Individual nursing measures can be selectively resolved by drawing a single line through them and entering the resolution date. All nursing measures may be discontinued using a bracket ([  ]) with date. Generally, if a nursing diagnosis is resolved and then reactivated, the entire problem is restated on the Kardex in another location. This is a simple mechanism to ensure that care is regularly reviewed and updated. All one has to do is compare the dates in the INITIATED and EVALUATED columns with today's date to determine if care is up-to-date or outdated. This is a perfect illustration of "built-in accountability." The same concepts apply to the standard care statements although the style is different.

**To make sure the staff uses standards of care properly,** consider them tools—all all tools require written guidelines. A complete set of guidelines addressing the details of selecting, implementing, evaluating, and documenting standards of care must be developed in participation with the staff and used as a basis for educating all nurses about their responsibilities. One thirty minute review based on the verbal word is totally inadequate because words are soon forgotten. In a short time, without a legitimate set of guidelines for direction, staff will be "doing their own thing" or nothing at all. Also, new staff coming into the system will not be properly oriented to standards. Potential problems must be worked out to the last detail. Consider these points as part of guidelines development:

1. Are the standards of care permanent parts of the chart or discarded?

2. Who is responsible for choosing these? How soon after admission should this be done?

3. How many standards of care can be used on one patient at a time? If restricted, does this apply to protocols?

4. Where will the standards of care be located while in effect for the patient? Who puts them there and removes them?

5. Who is responsible for individualizing them? Exactly how is this done?

6. Who is responsible for updating them and how?

7. How are the standards stored on the unit for easy access? Who maintains this?

8. What is the mechanism for altering the standard of care or protocol if it conflicts with professional nursing judgment or additional measures are required?

9. If you delete some aspect of care, should it be penciled out or permanently removed with a highlighter?

10. Will the nursing Kardex indicate which standard of care and protocols are in effect? How else will the regular nursing care Kardex be used? Should it be eliminated altogether?

11. How will the standards of care be documented?

## Documenting Standards

There are really two issues here: how to document standards and how standards can improve documentation. Briefly, traditional documentation has mandated that nursing notes contain all aspects of patient status and care given. We have had no choice but to write it all down—item by item and line by line both in nursing notes and on endless flowsheets. As soon as we think we've got a handle on it, another legal issue or third party payer says we have to record some other detail and so we expand our forms to incorporate it. And so it goes, until staff members are caught in the "Catch 22" situation of excessive charting demands and limited time. Nursing notes have grown in quantity but not necessarily in quality. Reams of repetitive assessment data and random details of care fill the papers.

Standards can greatly improve nursing record keeping by eliminating line item charting in notes and flow sheets, and documenting according to standards. By leaving the details in the standards of care and protocols, a single "Standards Documentation Flowsheet" can be used to record the majority of nursing care given. Then the nursing progress record can be limited to what is often omitted from nursing notations today—**evaluation of effectiveness of care in terms of patient response.** This would cut documentation time to a minimum, which will delight the staff; improve the content of what is charted, which will impress physicians and nurse managers; use documentation records more efficiently, which should make the medical records folks happy; and most important, reflect more of what is really taking place at the bedside, which will satisfy professional, legal, and financial requirements as well as quality assurance concerns.

The sample "Standards Documentation Flowsheet" (figure 10-1) is simple in design and use but a complete reflection of what the patient required and received. The guidelines for such a tool would direct the nurse to enter the standard of care being used by title on one side and initial each shift that she carried out the care as stated for the activated problems. A circled initial would indicate an exception or modification and refer the reader to an explanation in the nursing progress records. A single summation narrative or SOAP note at the end of the shift would be used to evaluate the patient's response to the plan in relation to defined outcome standards. The other side of the sheet would list each Protocol implemented by title, showing shift and date initiated and discontinued. Again initials for the shift would validate implementation with circled initials reflecting a problem or exception and a special nursing progress record notation for explanation. The shift summation would contain an evaluative statement about patient response to each protocol implemented during the shift.

## FIGURE 10-1

### STANDARDS DOCUMENTATION
### FLOWSHEET

**Front of page**

| STANDARD OF CARE (SCP/SCS) TITLE | Date | | | Date | | | Date | | | Date | | | Date | | | Date | | | Date | | | Date | | |
|---|---|---|---|---|---|---|---|---|---|---|---|---|---|---|---|---|---|---|---|---|---|---|---|---|
| | D | E | N | D | E | N | D | E | N | D | E | N | D | E | N | D | E | N | D | E | N | D | E | N |
| | | | | | | | | | | | | | | | | | | | | | | | | |
| | | | | | | | | | | | | | | | | | | | | | | | | |
| | | | | | | | | | | | | | | | | | | | | | | | | |
| | | | | | | | | | | | | | | | | | | | | | | | | |
| | | | | | | | | | | | | | | | | | | | | | | | | |

**Back of page**

| PROTOCOL TITLE | Date | | | Date | | | Date | | | Date | | | Date | | | Date | | | Date | | | Date | | |
|---|---|---|---|---|---|---|---|---|---|---|---|---|---|---|---|---|---|---|---|---|---|---|---|---|
| | D | E | N | D | E | N | D | E | N | D | E | N | D | E | N | D | E | N | D | E | N | D | E | N |
| | | | | | | | | | | | | | | | | | | | | | | | | |
| | | | | | | | | | | | | | | | | | | | | | | | | |
| | | | | | | | | | | | | | | | | | | | | | | | | |
| | | | | | | | | | | | | | | | | | | | | | | | | |
| | | | | | | | | | | | | | | | | | | | | | | | | |
| | | | | | | | | | | | | | | | | | | | | | | | | |

SIGNATURE VALIDATION: (Place signature and initials in the appropriate columns.)

| SIGNATURE | INITIALS | SIGNATURE | INITIALS | SIGNATURE | INITIALS |
|---|---|---|---|---|---|
| | | | | | |
| | | | | | |
| | | | | | |
| | | | | | |
| | | | | | |

These issues also apply to protocols.

Finally, to ensure long term effectiveness a **monitoring system for accountability** must be developed and integrated into the daily activities of the nursing unit, supervision activities, and unit-based quality assurance measures. This should include various checks to validate that the standards of care (and protocols) are being used. For example, when the Kardexes are used at report, charge nurses should be alert that the standards are in use; patient care rounds should focus on which standards are in use and how effectively they are being implemented; care conferences should focus on application and effectiveness of the standards; monthly staff meetings should denote a set time for standards review; general chart documentation audits should be done as well as specific observation reviews to determine the degree of compliance and effectiveness. The appropriate use of standards should be part of the unit's performance standards for the staff and built into the performance appraisal system.

Let's pull it all together with one last example. Let's say you've admitted an 86 year old lady from home with a fractured right hip sustained by a fall. It is 10:00 AM and she is scheduled for the OR for internal fixation that evening. She will be maintained in traction until that time. Her history includes CHF for which she takes daily Digitalis and Lasix. After you get her into bed, you would:

Action 1: Complete nursing data base and admission assessment.

Action 2: Pull the "SCP on Fractured Hip," individualizing it as needed.

Action 3: Pull the protocols as directed by the SCP—"Traction Protocol" and "Immobility Protocol."

Action 4: Pull any other protocols needed to support this patient's care— "Pre-Op Protocol" to prepare her for the OR.

Action 5: Add a nursing diagnosis on the patient's Kardex reflecting the secondary problem of CHF and critical measures to be carried out. The "CHF" SCP could serve as a reference for essential care. Usually the entire "CHF" SCP is unnecessary because it is designed for the patient whose primary problem is heart failure.

On the 3-11 shift, when the patient is returned from surgery, your evening co-worker would discontinue the traction and pre-op protocols. The "Fractured Hip SCP" and "Immobility Protocol" would remain in effect and the "Post-op Protocol" initiated. Let's assume that the next 48 hours go well, healing is progressing; no infection or immobility problems occur; physical activities are gradually increasing. However, the patient is losing weight and refusing to eat despite all nursing and dietary efforts. She is also anemic. The physician orders three units of packed cells to be administered on this third day post-op and tube feedings to be started. The "Blood Products Protocol" and "Tube Feeding Protocol" would now be initiated. The "Immobility Protocol" could be discontinued as soon as the patient is spending more than 50 percent of her time out of bed. This example shows how much time is saved by selecting and using standards as opposed to writing everything out from scratch. Quality care is being delivered and while the Standard of Care usually remains for the duration of the patient's stay, the protocols are flexible, starting and stopping as the nursing staff assess the patient's needs and modify the care accordingly. Finally, the Kardex is used to reflect individualized specific problems while the existing standards of care and protocols deal with the routine needs.

We've now climbed two of the three steps in the hierarchial Marker Model—structure standards and process standards. The top step—outcome standards—is the culmination of your standards development project.

# UNIT V: Outcome Standards

## Reaching the Apex

Outcome standards specify the results to be achieved through implementing structure and process standards. Written in the format of goal statements, they are located at the apex of the Marker Model because they are the most sophisticated of all standards. They stand atop both structure and process standards and rightfully so, since policies, job descriptions, performance standards, procedures, protocols, guidelines, and standards of care are all means for achieving positive results in patient care. Defining those positive results is what outcome standards are about.

# Chapter 11:   Specifying Outcomes

## USING OUTCOME STANDARDS

Outcome standards apply in four situations:

- Staff development,
- Patient education,
- Quality assurance,
- Care planning.

In the first two circumstances, you are trying to change behavior through education. So your outcome standards should specify the behaviors you want to see. These outcome standards are really teaching goals. Whenever you teach something, you begin with statements of your goals, proceed with content development, then define the methods to be used to achieve the goals. The outcome, in turn, reflects your success or failure and is used to measure results in the learner. This applies equally to both staff and patients. When a nurse manager identifies knowledge and skill deficits in her staff, she plans outcome directed learning activities to correct those deficiencies. For example, if the staff needs to become proficient at caring for colostomy patients, she would develop a learning session on the topic. The outcome standards for the program might be:

At the end of the colostomy review, the learner will be able to:

1. Identify the three types of ostomy appliances most often used at this hospital.
2. State the circumstances for which each type of appliance is recommended.
3. Carry out the "Protocol for Management of the Colostomy Patient."
4. Apply a karaya ring properly.
5. Discuss content and methodology in the "Protocol for Teaching Colostomy Patients."
6. Irrigate a colostomy according to procedure.

Outcome standards can also be developed by the nurse manager to correct performance deficiencies by incorporating a performance standard into a staff goal. These outcome standards tend to direct future performance rather than just state expected behaviors from a single learning session. They are usually written mutually by the manager and staff member at a coaching session or annual performance appraisal interview. Examples of outcome standards for staff development are:

> To become more proficient in starting peripheral IVs, John will start a line successfully in four different patients (including one emergency) within the next 6 weeks.

> To improve her organizational skills, Pam will keep an assignment worksheet, delegate specified taskes to nursing assistants, and reduce overtime use to once per pay period.

So outcome standards can serve as a focus for planning, implementing, and evaluating learning activities for both patients and staff, and also promote staff development.

Next, outcome standards assist in quality assurance activities. The fundamental purpose of quality assurance is to ensure safe and effective patient care by validating compliance to nursing standards. Outcome standards can serve as the basis for such evaluation. The methods, mechanisms, and tools that you use on your unit to evaluate patient care are directed at either structure, process, or outcome review. Structure review looks at compliance to your policies and how well structure standards contribute to an efficient nursing system. Process review determines how consistently and accurately nurses carry out predefined actions and the degree to which patients are receiving that care, in other words, compliance to process standards. Outcome reviews look only at the patient and determine whether he did or did not achieve the goals defined in the outcome standards. Unless outcome standards are predetermined and available, there is no basis for evaluating ultimate results of structure and process standards.

Finally, outcome standards are used in planning patient care. Consider the nursing process:

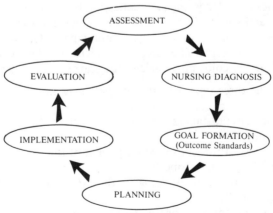

Assessment leads to identifying nursing diagnoses which leads to specifying outcome standards, in the format of goals. Outcome standards produce the plan for implementation. Evaluation completes the cycle and resolves the nursing diagnosis or leads to re-assessment and continuation of the process. Outcome standards provide the critical step between gathering and synthesizing information and actually using it to define nursing actions. This linkage of the problem and the plan is essential. Outcome standards give the plan direction and serve as the basis for its evaluation. To omit them is to violate nursing process.

## STYLE OF OUTCOME STANDARDS

To facilitate process and outcome reviews, there are two styles of Outcome Standards—nursing goals and patient outcomes. Nursing goals specify what nursing is to achieve. They determine the nature, extent, and content of nursing care. To write nursing goals, you would use **action verbs** such as reduce, restore, eliminate, maintain, minimize, observe, prevent, and promote. These verbs and the accompanying content provide direction for nursing actions and facilitate process review. The following statements are examples of nursing goals:

1. **Prevent** infection at the surgical site.
2. **Prevent** atelectasis in the initial 48 hours of bedrest postop.
3. **Minimize** further tissue deterioration at the wound site.
4. **Eliminate** risk of self injury during and after seizure activity.
5. **Reduce** dependency on IV narcotics for pain control.
6. **Promote** full ROM of affected right upper and lower extremities.

As discussed previously, the ill-defined and subjective phrase "short term goals" is obsolete and should not be used. Nursing goals can replace it.

Patient outcomes specify what the patient is to achieve. Often more sophisticated than nursing goals, patient outcomes are statements of condition written on three levels:

- **Physiological Outcomes** define a realistic level of physical health to be achieved by the patient.
- **Psychological Outcomes** define a realistic level of coping state and emotional well-being to be achieved by the patient.
- **Cognitive Outcomes** define a realistic level of knowledge that will allow the patient to take care of himself to the extent that he is able.

To write a patient outcome begin with "The patient will . . . ." Add the action verb such as: demonstrate (show and tell), achieve, accomplish, sustain, or maintain. Then complete the statement with the desired end. Be sure that the action statement describes an overt behavior. Since most all patient problems can be categorized as physical, psychological (emotional/spiritual), or self care requirements, the patient outcome statements will relate to the category of problem. Examples of patient outcomes are:

1. The patient's wound will heal.
2. The patient will maintain effective ventilation during the high-risk postop period.

3. The patient will achieve tissue granulation at the wound site.
4. The patient will be free of preventable physical injuries during and after seizure activity.
5. The patient will achieve his acceptable level of comfort on oral analgesics.
6. The patient will demonstrate effective use of his right side for ADL.

## COMPARING NURSING GOALS AND PATIENT OUTCOMES

### Nursing Goals

1. **Prevent** infection at the surgical site.
2. **Prevent** atelectasis in the initial 48 hours of bedrest postop.
3. **Mimimize** further tissue deterioration at the wound site.
4. **Eliminate** risk of self injury during and after seizure activity.
5. **Reduce** dependency on IV narcotics for pain control.
6. **Promote** full ROM of affected right upper and lower extremities.

### Patient Outcomes

1. The patient's wound will heal.
2. The patient will maintain effective ventilation during the high-risk postop period.
3. The patient will achieve tissue granulation of the wound site.
4. The patient will be free of preventable physical injuries during and after seizure activity.
5. The patient will achieve his acceptable level of comfort on oral analgesics.
6. The patient will demonstrate effective use of right side for ADL.

In reading over both sets of examples, note how each nursing goal was extended into a patient outcome to reflect the final condition in the patient. By designing care to meet the nursing goal, the patient outcome should be facilitated. For instance, in nursing goal number 3, nursing measures taken to reduce dependency on IV narcotics should assist the patient to be comfortable on oral medications only. In nursing goal number 6, nursing measures taken to promote full ROM of affected extremities should result in the patient's ability to use them for self care. The differentiation is important because some nurses think that nursing goals and patient outcomes are the same thing. **Nursing goals are written for the care giver while patient outcomes are written for the care recipient.**

The patient outcomes provide the basis for development of outcome criteria to perform outcome reviews. Much has been written about the importance of time frames in outcome standards. Note that the above outcomes do not contain absolute time frames. This is because absolute time frames may not be achievable due to events beyond the nurse's control. Since the average hospital stay is now between four and seven days, obviously the outcomes should be accomplished before discharge. If they cannot, the patient is being discharged regardless, due to economic realities. Failure to meet patient outcomes today means transfer to another longer term care facility and/or home health care assistance. Also, in the suggested Kardex and standard care plan style, the initiated, evaluated, and resolved date columns can be used very effectively to evaluate the patient's progress each twenty-four hours toward resolution of the nursing diagnosis and accomplishment of the desired state. This is a much more reasonable way to use outcome standards. Arbitrary time frames can be restrictive and unrealistic. They often have to be altered, thus giving nurses an unnecessary sense of failure.

The phrase "long-term goals" is an inappropriate as "short-term goals." Eliminate it from Kardexes and care planning activities. **Use "patient outcomes" instead.**

In addition to short and long goals, some nursing Kardexes also contain spaces for "teaching objectives" and "discharge criteria." As emphasized previously, when patient outcomes are written to specify physical, emotional, and educational needs of the patient in context with appropriate nursing diagnoses teaching objectives are no longer necessary. Since patient outcomes become discharge criteria for that patient population, this section can also be removed. Well developed outcome standards can prevent duplication of writing efforts and shorten the Kardex. Thus we see once more how nursing standards can help nurses work smarter, not harder.

## INCORPORATING OUTCOME STANDARDS

Two legitimate places exist in your standards for outcome standards. Both are process: the format of **Teaching Protocols** and the format of **Standards of Care.** This is consistent with the use of outcome standards in education and care planning. While outcomes are the third and final type of standard, they really can't exist in isolation. Structure standards stand alone because they are so important. Process standards stand alone because they are so extensive and comprehensive. **However outcome standards must be incorporated into other standards,** namely, teaching protocols and standards of care. To put them in procedures, protocols (other than educational ones), or guidelines is unnecessary and time consuming. If you look back at the styles of these formats, you'll see "purpose" instead of outcomes. That is all that is necessary because the focus of these three formats is process while the focus of Teaching Protocols and Standards of Care is both process and outcome.

In relation to teaching protocols, the outcome standards are placed at the beginning to serve as a basis for content to be taught. Since health care teaching is done to promote a physical and emotional wellbeing in the patient as well as prepare him for self care, an outcome statement is written at each level. Review the example of the "Colostomy Teaching Protocol." The patient outcomes begin with the physiologic domain and progress through the psychologic and cognitive.

| HOSPITAL | INITIATED | DISCONTINUED |
|---|---|---|
| DEPARTMENT OF NURSING | DATE _____ | DATE _____ |
| | TIME _____ | TIME _____ |
| | RN _____ | RN _____ |

**TEACHING PROTOCOL**
**FOR:** *NEW COLOSTOMY PATIENT*

PURPOSE: To outline nursing responsibility in patient education of a patient/SO with a new colostomy.

LEVEL:     Independent (requires nursing order only)

CONTENT:

| OUTCOME STANDARDS: | DATE MET/SIGN |
|---|---|
| PHYSIOLOGIC: ▶ The colostomy patient will achieve and maintain normal bowel function through effective self care. | |
| PYSCHOLOGIC: ▶ The colostomy patient will demonstrate an attitude of acceptance of modified life style (altered bowel function and body image). | |
| COGNITIVE: ▶ The colostomy patient will demonstrate the ability to manage his colostomy independently (or with SO assistance). | |

| Information to be Delivered | Methodology | Taught By/Date | Patient/SO Response |
|---|---|---|---|
| | | | |

Then the teaching protocol outlines what content will be taught to accomplish the stated outcomes as well as the methods for doing so (visual aids, charts, films, booklets, and so forth). Final columns call for date, responsible person actively conveying the material, and patient response. Note that beside each outcome standard is a small section for "Date Met." This allows the team member to verify that the teaching protocol has been effective and the patient outcomes have been achieved. In using this tool, all team members can tell at a glance where each patient is in his learning and when nursing responsibilities are complete.

In standards of care, you have a choice as to which type of outcome standards you write. If you develop an SCS, you would write three general outcomes for the patient population in the DRG—physiologic, psychologic, and cognitive. If you elect to go with an SCP and use the two or four column approach, you would write both nursing goals and patient outcomes. But if you choose the three column approach, you would write only patient outcomes, because outcome standards are necessary to outcome review, they always take priority.

This example shows the most sophisticated standard of care using all four columns. Outcome standards in the style of a SCP address each nursing diagnosis in terms of both nursing achievements and patient results. Note the flow of the nursing process from initiation through evaluation to resolution.

**HOSPITAL**

**DEPARTMENT OF NURSING**

STANDARD OF CARE (SCP)
ON PATIENTS WITH: *Carotid Endarterectomy*

INITIATED ▢  DISCONTINUED ▢

DATE _____   DATE _____
TIME _____   TIME _____
RN _____     RN _____

| NURSING DIAGNOSIS / PATIENT CARE PROBLEM | NURSING GOALS | PATIENT OUTCOME | EVALUATED DATE | RN | NURSING INTERVENTIONS | RESOLVED DATE | RN |
|---|---|---|---|---|---|---|---|
| INITIATED: DATE / RN | | | | | | | |
| 1. Pain op site | • Minimize post op pain | • The patient will achieve comfort level conducive to stable vital signs and compliance with role. | | | | | |
| 2. Potential for hemorrhage at suture/graft site and decreased cerebral perfusion | • Observe for evidence of loss integrity of graft | • The patient will maintain effective cerebral perfusion and stable neurologic status. | | | | | |
| 3. Potential for airway obstruction/respiratory insufficiency/dependency on mechanical ventilator | • Assess adequacy of ventilation/perfusion and need for $O_2$ support/airway augmentation | • The patient will achieve stable ventilatory status as evidenced by stable ABGs. | | | | | |
| 4. Potential for unstable/abnormal heart rate, rhythm, and blood pressure/dependency on titrated medications | • Maintain stable CV status re: B/P, HR and rhythm | • The patient will achieve adequate CO to maintain effective tissue perfusion. | | | | | |
| 5. Potential wound infection | • Prevent post op wound infection | • The patient will achieve a normal healing wound post op. | | | | | |
| 6. Potential fear/anxiety 2° unknown | • Observe for excessive anxiety and promote a level of understanding of events and calmness during early post op state | • The patient will overcome post op anxiety and exhibit early positive coping ability to imposed limitations. | | | | | |

In this standard of care using the three column approach, the outcome standards are limited to patient outcomes only. There is still an outcome standard for each stated nursing diagnosis and the flow from initiated through evaluation to resolution.

| | | | | | DISCONTINUED |
|---|---|---|---|---|---|
| | HOSPITAL | | | | DATE _____ |
| | DEPARTMENT OF NURSING | | | | TIME _____ |
| | | | | | RN _____ |

STANDARD OF CARE (SCP) ON THE PATIENT
WITH: *Acute Myocardial Infarction*

| INITIATED | | NURSING DIAGNOSIS | OUTCOME STANDARDS (PATIENT OUTCOME) | EVALUATED | | NURSING INTERVENTIONS | RESOLVED | |
|---|---|---|---|---|---|---|---|---|
| DATE | RN | | | DATE | RN | | DATE | RN |
| | | 1. Chest pain 2° accumulated cellular metabolites | • Patient will achieve a pain free state. | | | | | |
| | | 2. ↓CO leading to potential poor tissue perfusion (forward failure) | • Patient will maintain physiologic tissue perfusion. | | | | | |
| | | 3. ↑LVEDP leading to potential pulmonary congestion (backward failure) | • Patient will achieve stable ABG's using normal breathing patterns with appropriate energy expenditure. | | | | | |
| | | 4. Potential for major/lethal cardiac arrhythmias | • Patient will maintain a physiologic rate and rhythm to achieve effective CO. | | | | | |
| | | 5. Potential for fear/anxiety 2° condition and prognosis | • Patient will achieve a calm, relaxed emotional state supported by his significant others. | | | | | |
| | | 6. Potential knowledge deficit 2° to CAD and self care post MI | • Patient and SO will demonstrate self care skills required for discharge. | | | | | |

In this standard of care using the two column approach, the SCP allows both nursing goals and patient outcomes but places them at the bottom of the form. The goals and outcomes are directed at the DRG (patient population) and have a relationship to the nursing diagnoses but are not necessarily related to each nursing diagnostic statement. The tool allows evaluation of the goals and notation of resolution of each patient outcome.

HOSPITAL
DEPARTMENT OF NURSING

| INITIATED | DISCONTINUED |
|---|---|
| DATE _____ | DATE _____ |
| TIME _____ | TIME _____ |
| RN _____ | RN _____ |

STANDARD OF CARE (SCP) ON THE PATIENT
WITH: *Cholecystectomy with CBD exploration*

| INITIATED DATE | RN | NURSING DIAGNOSIS | NURSING INTERVENTIONS | DISCONTINUED DATE | RN |
|---|---|---|---|---|---|
| | | 1. Altered physiologic condition 2° post op state. | | | |
| | | 2. Post-op pain and splinting 2° high abdominal incision and extensive surgical manipulation. | | | |
| | | 3. Potential for complications 2° T tube (skin breakdown, dislodgement, blockage). | | | |
| | | 4. Potential complications 2° GI intubation. | | | |
| | | 5. Potential fear and anxiety 2° condition and prognosis. | | | |
| | | 6. Potential for knowledge deficit for self care post discharge. | | | |

| NURSING GOALS | EVALUATED DATE | RN | PATIENT OUTCOMES | RESOLVED DATE | RN |
|---|---|---|---|---|---|
| 1. Prevent post-op complications of fluid & electrolyte imbalance, pneumonia, and paralytic ileus. | | | 1. Patient will achieve and maintain a stable post op state free of complications. | | |
| 2. Maintain post op comfort. | | | 2. Patient will achieve a comfort state which facilitates his cooperation in physical activity and pulmonary care. | | |
| 3. Prevent complications of T-tube and GI intubation. | | | 3. The patient will maintain stable fluid and electrolyte balance. | | |
| 4. Minimize unnecessary psychological discomfort. | | | 4. The patient will resume physiologic GI function. | | |
| 5. Promote progressive physical self care and educate patient for home care post discharge. | | | 5. Patient will assume self care responsibility on unit with SO assistance and demonstrate knowledge of information in "Post Op Teaching Protocol". | | |

Finally, this example demonstrates how outcome standards would be written in a standard of care in the style of SCS. Note the simple columns for initiating and discontinuing problems and care measures. Note also the "Date Met/ Signature" column to indicate accomplishment.

**HOSPITAL**
DEPARTMENT OF NURSING

| INITIATED | DISCONTINUED |
|---|---|
| DATE _____ | DATE _____ |
| TIME _____ | TIME _____ |
| RN _____ | RN _____ |

STANDARD OF CARE (SCS) ON THE PATIENT
WITH: *Congestive Heart Failure*

| OUTCOME STANDARDS: | DATE MET/SIGN |
|---|---|
| PHYSIOLOGIC OUTCOME: ▶ The patient will achieve adequate cardiac output to minimize symptoms and carry out ADL. | |
| PSYCHOLOGIC OUTCOME: ▶ The patient will experience minimal anxiety due to pathologic condition and demonstrate acceptance of living with chronic cardiac disability. | |
| COGNITIVE OUTCOME: ▶ The patient will explain "failure state" and demonstrate self care skills. | |

| INITIATED | | SUBJECT HEADINGS | NURSING INTERVENTIONS | DISCONTINUED | |
|---|---|---|---|---|---|
| DATE | RN | | | DATE | RN |
| | | ASSESSMENT | 1. Assess systems for evidence of progressive CHF each shift to include:<br> ▲ Apical/radial rate for one minute for rate/regularity; neck veins for ↑JVP.<br> ▲ B/P (position of comfort).<br> ▲ Respiratory rate and character (degree of effort, use of accessory muscles, orthopnea, pillows required).<br> ▲ Posterior chest auscultation for rales/rhonchi/wheezing (inspir./expir.).<br> ▲ Abdomen for distention, BS, RUQ pain.<br> ▲ Lower extremities (hands and dependent body parts) for presence and degree of edema (1, 2, 3 plus).<br> ▲ Presence of calf tenderness. | | |
| | | FLUID BALANCE | 2. Weight patient daily and record on I/O record.<br> 3. Report positive fluid balance (>1 liter/24 hrs.)<br> 4. Place on I/O q 8 hours if positive fluid balance is evident; if UP less than sufficient; if 3 + edema develops; if pulmonary edema develops.<br> 5. Place on I/O if on IVs (use only micro-drips and 500 cc bottles; all IVs to be on controllers).<br> 6. Discuss with MD the ordering of electrolytes q 48 hours if patient is newly placed on diuretics or if output >2000/24 hours or >1000cc/shift. | | |

# MEASURING OUTCOME STANDARDS—
## DIFFERENTIATING STANDARDS AND CRITERIA

We have seen the different ways in which outcome standards can be written and have briefly discussed their use in education and evaluation of care. Obviously, if outcome standards are to be used in quality assurance activities, they must be measurable. All the outcome standards used in the examples—both nursing goals and patient outcomes—are easily measurable after criteria for measurement have been written! Generally standards and measuring criteria are not written simultaneously. This would make standards of development much too complicated and tedious! Standards are developed first. Measuring criteria are written at the time you want to practice formal quality assurance. Criteria for evaluating effectiveness of care or patient accomplishment evolve from the Standards. Criteria are key elements of care which are selected to reflect compliance or non-compliance to a standard. Criteria must be objective and participatively developed. They contain five parts:

- the element of care desired,
- the frequency desired,
- the desired compliance factor,
- any predefined exceptions to the care,
- what precisely demonstrates compliance.

Criteria development requires time and thought. A specific criteria development tool facilitates their development but that is another topic entirely. Suffice it to say, standards development and criteria writing for measurement of care through QA activities are two closely related but rather different activities.

# UNIT VI: Standards Development

# Chapter 12:   Putting It All Together

Before you can begin planning your standards development project, you must feel comfortable with the content presented thus far. This chapter helps you solidify your working understanding of the basic tenets of the Marker Model and your ability to utilize the Model appropriately.

**Exercise 1** helps you brainstorm your way through a problem using standards. You become familiar with using the standards problem-solving approach as the basis for identifying those areas in need of standards.

**Exercise 2** perfects your ability to look at a problem, identify what type and format of standard is required, what content should be included, and where the standard fits into your unit manual.

**Exercise 3** focuses on structure and strengthens your skills to classify specific unit topics according to the 9 elements of unit structure. It helps you to differentiate between issues that should appear in the body of your policies and those which should be addressed in addenda.

**Exercises 4 and 5** test your proficiency in analyzing a procedure and a protocol according to the Model's approach for procedure and protocol development to identify strengths, weaknesses, and your suggestions for improvement.

**Exercise 6** refines your skills for classifying process issues into one of the six formats. **Exercise 7** challenges you to identify which protocols are priority protocols for specific standards of care.

These exercises help you identify your own strengths and weaknesses in using the Marker Model. They also provide the basic skills you need to begin work on your standards development project. Your degree of success with these application exercises will determine which pieces of the model you can begin to tackle immediately and which pieces will require more concentrated study.

## EXERCISE #1: PROBLEM SOLVING

Instructions: Read the following hypothetical situation and answer the questions. Compare your answers to the discussion on page 147.

You are reviewing recent quality assurance activities on your unit: two patient care audits, several concurrent monitors on pertinent unit issues, a documentation review, care conference reports, and supervisory rounds reports. Your rounds in particular reflect a consistent problem with inadequate nutritional support in your patient population. You note a pattern in this deficiency as you scan your QA Quarterly Report. As you critique the issue of nutritional care on your unit, you conclude that the staff members are not:

- including nutritional assessment on admission assessments or periodically throughout the hospitalization.

- placing patients on daily weights or calorie counts when it becomes obvious that intake is inadequate.

- noting the impact of limited nutrition on mental status, muscle strength, or wound healing.

- utilizing the dietitians to their full potential in unit consultation or consistently inviting them to unit care conferences.

- seeking information or literature on patient nutritional support.

- consistently evaluating effectiveness of alternate feeding mechanisms (TPN, tube feedings).

- pursuing discussion and collaboration on nutritional support with the medical staff.

- helping patients who require assistance to complete their menu selections.

- addressing nutritional limitations in care planning or care conferences.

You are especially concerned because your patients are generally older, chronically ill, and have a longer duration of stay due to multiple systems pathologies:

A. What is the first question you should ask and the first action you should take?

B. In reviewing your unit manual, you find the following protocols:

- Alteration in Nutrition/Elimination Status
- Total Parenteral Nutrition
- Tube Feeding
- Lipid Infusion
- Nutritional Support

1. What conclusion can you draw from this information?

    2. What is the next question you should ask?

    3. What actions would you take in response to answering question 2?

C. Suppose, however, that in reviewing your unit manual, you do not find specific protocols addressing patients' nutritional needs.

    1. What can you conclude from this and what should you do about it?

    2. List the steps you would take to correct the problem you've identified.

Discussion: Absence of adequate nutritional support is the result of the problem this manager perceives, not really the problem. But, exactly what is the problem?

A. First, ask yourself "DO I have a well written standard addressing nutritional management of my patients?" To assure yourself of the answer, review your unit standards manual.

B. 1. Based on your review you can conclude yes, standards do exist relative to this area.

    2. The question now becomes, "WHO is non-compliant and why?"

    3. You have now pinpointed your real problem—standards are present and adequately identify what constitutes nutritional management of your patients, but staff are not adhering to them. Thus your first task is to "audit the noncompliance." This should be done by sitting down with a group of staff members, reviewing the nutritional protocols, pulling essential criteria from the standards, and collecting process data observing both specific staff members and patient situations. This participative quality assurance will give you and your staff a clear picture of non-compliance by answering precisely which staff members are following the protocols and which ones are not. The compliant staff should be acknowledged and given positive feedback. The non-compliant staff should be counseled and directly involved in the corrective action, both its planning and execution. Corrective actions for non-compliance usually involve in-service education and a review of activities to increase staff knowledge and awareness of a particular aspect of patient care or staff performance. Monitoring actions would then be set up to make sure that the problem is resolved and stays that way.

C. 1. Obviously, in this instance, standards do not exist. You now know the precise nature of your deficit. The problem is the lack of definition of what nurses should do and what patients should receive relative to nutritional support. Now you know exactly what you need to do for corrective action—write one!

    2. There are five critical steps in writing a standard. The first step requires *seeking input* from persons knowledgeable about the topic, persons who will be involved in implementing the standard, and finally persons with power to change the present situation. The final draft

involves step 2, *gaining approval*. This is critical to giving the new standard the credibility and clout needed for successful implementation. The approved standard is now ready to be presented to the staff (step 3). *Educating staff* involves not only reviewing the content of the standard with the staff but also specifying how the new standard will be used on the unit. Once the staff is knowledgeable, step 4, *implementing the standard*, must be actively pursued. Implementation involves all levels of management creating mechanisms for staff compliance.

Finally, *monitoring results*, step 5, is reviewing both the use of the Standard and its effectiveness in patient care. Here monitoring refers to short and long term QA activities. This is the last essential managerial function to evaluate whether the standard has been successful in resolving the initial patient care problem. Success would be measured by any one of the following: absence of the problem in the future, reduction in the frequency of the problem, or a decrease in the negative impact of the problem on the system, staff, or patients.

If you need more practice with this exercise, review the content on problem-solving in chapter one and study the standards problem-solving flowchart. If you answered the above questions correctly, you are ready to assess your unit or department to identify what problems exist and what to do about them.

## EXERCISE #2: STANDARDS MATCHING

Once you decide to write a standard, it is essential to determine both the TYPE and the FORMAT of standard you need to correct your identified problem. This exercise is designed to give you practice in making decisions about writing your standards using the Marker Model.

Keep these helpful hints in mind as you work on this exercise:

- IF IT IS NOT A NURSING RESPONSIBILITY DEFINED BY THE LAW, ANA, JCAH, OR YOUR MANAGEMENT VALUES, IT DOES NOT GO INTO THE JOB DESCRIPTION.

- IF IT IS NOT A PART OF THE JOB DESCRIPTION, IT DOES NOT GO INTO A PERFORMANCE STANDARD.

- IF IT IS NOT A PSYCHOMOTOR SKILL (In/Out . .Up/Down . . . On/Off . . Start/Stop . . . ) THEN IT DOES NOT GO INTO A PROCEDURE.

- IF IT IS NOT AN ASPECT OF CARE AND MANAGEMENT OF A BROAD PROBLEM OR ISSUE IN FIVE CATEGORIES (Care of Patients on Non-invasive Equipment; Care of Patients on Invasive Equipment; Management of Therapeutic, Diagnostic, or Prophylactic Measures; Care of Problematic, Physiologic or Psychologic States; Interventions in Selected Nursing Diagnoses) THEN IT DOES NOT GO INTO A PROTOCOL.

- IF IT IS NOT A FORM OR TOOL FOR COMMUNICATION OR DOCUMENTATION, THEN IT DOES NOT GO INTO A GUIDELINE.

- IF IT IS NOT A DIAGNOSTIC PATIENT POPULATION (DRG), THEN IT DOES NOT GO INTO A STANDARD OF CARE.

Let's run through an example of how your thoughts should proceed before you begin:

| | |
|---|---|
| Issue: | Shift report. |
| Type of Standard? | |
| Your Thoughts: | This is an aspect of running the nursing unit; it is STRUCTURE. |
| Type of Format? | |
| Your Thoughts: | The format of structure is policy. I must have policy to define the parameters of shift report. |
| Suggested Content? | |
| Your Thoughts: | Who gives report? |
| | Who attends report? |
| | When is it given? |
| | How long should it be? |
| | Is it a general overview in a large group and then more detailed 1:1 bedside discussion or a detailed report for the entire staff? |
| | Is it taped or oral? |
| | Are walking rounds a part of it? |
| | Should this occur on all patients or just the most critical? |
| | What should the content be in order to make the most of the limited time? |
| | How will unit standards be integrated into shift report? |
| Location? | |
| Your Thoughts: | In reviewing the 9 elements of Unit structure, shift report is not part of the UNIT DESCRIPTION, PURPOSE, or OBJECTIVES. Neither is it relevant to ADMINISTRATION/ORGANIZATION, HOURS OF OPERATION, or USE OF THE NURSING UNIT. It doesn't fit into GOVERNING RULES either. But it does link in with the STAFFING section of my unit structure. The staffing element contains four components: Quantity, Levels, Delivery of Care Methodology, and Preparation. Delivery of Care Methodology contains these topics: method of care delivery; delivery system; assignment mechanisms, shift report routines; function of charge nurse; and accountability of non-professional staff members. My policy on shift report belongs in the staff- |

ing section of my unit manual under "Delivery of Care Methodology."

In a few minutes of structured brainstorming, you can lay the groundwork for your standards development by classifying issues and clarifying content.

Once you know the Model, the types, and formats, and content, you spend a minimal amount of time deciding what to do with an issue and a maximum amount of time getting it done!

Now you try it. These 16 topics are among the most common issues raised by groups of nurses across the country by nominal group process.

*Issues*

1. Temporary assignment of staff (floating),
2. Patient education
3. Assessment (patient assessment on admission and thereafter),
4. Nursing data base (admission nursing history and physical),
5. Discharge planning,
6. Competency (how to define and measure it),
7. Care planning,
8. AIDS,
9. Safety,
10. Chemotherapy,
11. Skin integrity,
12. Fetal monitoring,
13. Assaultive behavior,
14. Infection control,
15. Ventilator care,
16. Ventilator flow sheet,
17. Drawing ABGs.

Instructions:

From a staff or head nurse point of view in your specific nursing unit, look at these 17 issues and identify the type and format of standard that best matches the topic, outline potential content, and where to put the standard in your unit standards manual. Compare your answers to those that follow. Use the following chart for each issue:

| Issue | Type of Standard | Format of Standard | Suggested Content | Location |
|-------|------------------|--------------------|--------------------|----------|
|       |                  |                    |                    |          |

| Issue | Type of Standard | Format of Standard | Suggested Content | Location |
|---|---|---|---|---|
| TEMPORARY ASSIGNMENT OF STAFF (floating) | STRUCTURE | POLICY — Element VIII "Staffing" (under "Levels") | — Circumstances under which floats are sent to your unit;<br>— How they receive report, orientation, and assignments.<br>— How assignments are altered?<br>  — support measures for floats such as standards and supervision;<br>  — mechanisms to record float assignments for fairness and budgetary purposes. | STRUCTURE SECTION — Staffing Element VIII |
| PATIENT EDUCATION | PROCESS | PROTOCOL (specifically) TEACHING PROTOCOL + incorporate OUTCOME STANDARDS in the format of teaching goals; (see page xx) | — What outcome standards are to be achieved?<br>— What content is to be taught in relation to the educational issue and goals?<br>— What methods are to be used to teach, including 1:1, group, AV aids, testing, demonstration/patient feedback?<br>— How is education to be documented?<br>— What evidence will determine if learning has taken place? | PROCESS SECTION — Protocols tab (alphabetized) |
| ASSESSMENT (patient assessment on admission and thereafter) | PROCESS | PERFORMANCE STANDARDS | — What parameters constitute assessment?<br>— When must it be done and how frequently?<br>— How will it be recorded? | PROCESS SECTION Performance Standards tab |
| NURSING DATA BASE (admission nursing H/P) | PROCESS | GUIDELINES FOR NDB | — Is it a permanent or temporary part of chart?<br>— Where does it go in the record?<br>— Who fills it out and when?<br>— How is each line/box/entry to be completed?<br>— What should it look like when completed? | PROCESS SECTION Guidelines tab |

| Issue | Type of Standard | Format of Standard | Suggested Content | Location |
|---|---|---|---|---|
| DISCHARGE PLANNING | STRUCTURE | POLICY Element VII — "Use of Nursing Unit" (after admission routine/criteria/duration of stay are defined; discharge planning activities are discussed in the "Transfer/Discharge" section. | — Who does the discharge planning?<br>— When does it take place?<br>  — use of discharge planning rounds;<br>  — collaboration between physicians and nursing staff on patient status;<br>  — multidisciplinary focus;<br>  — documented evidence that patients are ready for discharge in relation to unit discharge criteria. | STRUCTURE SECTION — Use of Nursing Unit Element VII |
| COMPETENCY — How to define and measure? | STRUCTURE<br><br>and<br><br>PROCESS | POLICY Element VIII — "Staffing" (under "Preparation" after selection/hiring/orientation/special preparation/continuing education, is the content on validation of staff competency).<br><br>PERFORMANCE STANDARDS | — How and when is competency validation done? (address both cognitive and skill testing.)<br>— How and where are records kept?<br>— What is the staff's participation?<br>— What measures are in place to deal with poor staff results?<br>— How does this relate to QA and performance appraisal?<br><br>— What constitutes the manager's expectations of staff in relation to the patient population, acuity level of patients, and values of the nursing leadership?<br>— What broad responsibilities are outlined in the level Job Description and how do these relate to my specific unit staff?<br>  — list specific measurable behaviors required in relation to the 28 responsibilities of RN staff (see page xx). | STRUCTURE SECTION — Staffing Element VIII<br><br>PROCESS SECTION — Performance Standards tab |

| Issue | Type of Standard | Format of Standard | Suggested Content | Location |
|---|---|---|---|---|
| CARE PLANNING | PROCESS | PERFORMANCE STANDARDS | — What precisely is expected of the staff in terms of care planning?<br>— Who initiates care plans?<br>— How are they maintained, individualized/modified, and updated?<br>— How is implementation documented and evaluation of effectiveness reflected in the patient record? | PROCESS SECTION — Performance Standards tab |
| | | and<br><br>GUIDELINES | — How is the tool itself used (as part of the cardboard Kardex system or a separate piece of paper)?<br>— Is it a permanent part of the record/completed in pen or pencil?<br>— Exactly how is one completed and what goes into the various columns? | PROCESS SECTION — Guidelines tab |
| AIDS | PROCESS | STANDARD OF CARE (diagnostic patient population/DRG)<br>+<br>incorporate OUTCOME STANDARDS (in the format of patient outcomes). | — What are the key nursing diagnoses or patient care problems of patients with this pathology?<br>— What patient outcomes do the staff work toward?<br>— What specific nursing interventions must be carried out in relation to potential respiratory infection; cross contamination; skin lesions; blood dyscrasias, fear of impending death?<br>— What documentation is required? | PROCESS SECTION — Standards of Care tab |

| Issue | Type of Standard | Format of Standard | Suggested Content | Location |
|---|---|---|---|---|
| SAFETY | STRUCTURE | POLICY Element VII — "Governing Rules" (usually a broad statement and specific addenda) | — What issues present increased risk of patient/staff incidents and increased litigation possibilities? — include issues such as patient identification, medical administration, electrical safety, fall prevention, smoking regulations, staff identification, use of incident reports, side rails, safety straps, restraints, beds in low position, night lights. — address safety practices designed to minimize these. — documentation of safety events. — relationship to quality assurance monitoring on the unit. | STRUCTURE SECTION — Governing Rules Element VII |
| CHEMO-THERAPY | PROCESS | PROCEDURE and PROTOCOL | — How to mix, hang and discontinue from a skills standpoint. — Assessment factors/frequency; patient instruction; evaluating effectiveness; side effects/complications and nursing management of issues such as GI upset, hair loss, blood component suppression, altered body image, infection control measures. — documentation of patient response. — reportable conditions to physician. | PROCESS SECTION — Procedures tab PROCESS SECTION — Protocols tab |
| SKIN INTEGRITY | PROCESS | PROTOCOL | — Who are candidates for this protocol? — assessment of skin and potential breakdown areas; prophylactic measures, frequency, and evaluation? — additional nursing care measures for failure to prevent alteration in skin integrity (i.e., appearance of redness, excoriation, and frank decubitus). — documentation of events and effectiveness. | PROCESS SECTION — Protocols tab |

| Issue | Type of Standard | Format of Standard | Suggested Content | Location |
|---|---|---|---|---|
| FETAL MONITORING | PROCESS | PROCEDURE<br><br>and<br><br>PROTOCOL | — What psychomotor skill steps are followed in attaching the patient to external or internal fetal monitoring equipment?<br>— how to set alarms, load paper, produce printouts and check calibration.<br><br>— What assessment of the mother and fetus must take place and with what frequency?<br>— instruction to the patient.<br>— psychologic support.<br>— comfort measures.<br>— electrical safety concerns.<br>— precautions/complications.<br>— emergency measures for fetal distress indications.<br>— notification of the physician.<br>— documentation of observations and nursing actions. | PROCESS SECTION — Procedures tab<br><br>PROCESS SECTION — Protocols tab |
| ASSAULTIVE BEHAVIOR | PROCESS | PROTOCOL | — What constitutes assaultive behavior and requires use of this protocol?<br>— What assessments of patient behavior must take place and with what frequency?<br>— nursing management of offensive and dangerous behaviors including distance, touch, eye contact.<br>— limitations of patient privileges.<br>— staff approach/demeanor.<br>— isolation.<br>— evaluation of effectiveness.<br>— notification of physician.<br>— documentation of events. | PROCESS SECTION — Protocols tab |

| Issue | Type of Standard | Format of Standard | Suggested Content | Location |
|---|---|---|---|---|
| INFECTION CONTROL | STRUCTURE | POLICY Element VII — "Governing Rules" (usually a broad general statement and specific addenda) | — What specific situations on the unit create increased risk of infection/cross contamination related to geographics of unit?<br>— staff parameters, patient population/acuity,<br>— Measures taken to reduce risk.<br>— How do these relate to hospital and departmental measures? | STRUCTURE SECTION — Governing Rules Element VII |
| VENTILATOR CARE | PROCESS | PROTOCOL | — Ongoing assessment of patient and ventilator system:<br>— trouble shooting.<br>— potential complications and nursing management.<br>— comfort/communication measures.<br>— psychologic support.<br>— suctioning routines.<br>— diagnostic measures such as ABGs and chest xrays.<br>— evaluation of effectiveness of ventilator and nursing measures.<br>— reportable situations.<br>— essential documentation. | PROCESS SECTION — Protocols tab |
| VENTILATOR FLOWSHEET | PROCESS | GUIDELINES | Directions for completion of form in detail with examples of each section and then entire form in completed state. | PROCESS SECTION — Guidelines tab |
| DRAWING ABGs | STRUCTURE<br><br>PROCESS | POLICY Element IX — "Nursing Responsibilities"<br><br>PROCEDURE | — Address whether staff is permitted to carry out this controversial act in terms of aspiration from existing lines only or through arterial stick:<br>— Specify any requirements and restrictions, such as "no femoral punctures."<br>— Address education and credentialing measures.<br>— What is the precise technique used to obtain ABGs. | STRUCTURE SECTION — Nursing Responsibility Element IX<br>PROCESS SECTION— Procedures tab |

How did you do? Was there one type of Standard that you felt particularly comfortable or weak in? If so, that's natural. You need practice. You may wish to reread certain segments of the book to help you over the rough spots.

Those issues that you brainstormed correctly will provide the basis for writing some of your own standards. When you feel confident in this skill, use this approach to help you deal with issues that are specific to your particular unit. It will save you an inordinate amount of time and get your standards writing off on the right foot.

## EXERCISE #3: STRUCTURE MATCHING

Instructions: Read through this list of structure topics and identify which element of your unit structure is best suited to the information. Place the number of the structure element in the parentheses (see Table 3-3). All of the topics integrate into only one element of structure. Then determine whether the policy statements addressing the topic would more likely be in the main body of your structure or an addendum. (Remember that addenda are under separate tabs in your unit standards manual and are used to define content that is very specific, detailed, and changeable.) Compare your responses with those that follow.

| TOPICS | ELEMENT (number) | MAIN BODY ( ) | ADDENDUM ( ) |
|---|---|---|---|
| 1. nurses' limitations of practice. | | | |
| 2. relationship of unit with admitting office | | | |
| 3. bed size | | | |
| 4. narrative | | | |
| 5. preventing microshock hazards | | | |
| 6. equipment check frequency | | | |
| 7. orientation of unit personnel | | | |
| 8. relationship of unit to essential support services | | | |
| 9. role of charge nurse | | | |
| 10. use of nursing process on unit | | | |
| 11. accountability of LPN to RN staff | | | |
| 12. required continuing education activities | | | |
| 13. crash cart checklist | | | |
| 14. limitations of unit in dealing with patient populations and clinical issues | | | |
| 15. organizational chart for unit | | | |
| 16. replacement of broken equipment | | | |
| 17. infection control issues for unit | | | |

| TOPICS | ELEMENT (number) | MAIN BODY ( ) | ADDENDUM ( ) |
|---|---|---|---|
| 18. staffing patterns for the unit | | | |
| 19. discharge criteria | | | |
| 20. provision of hemodialysis to unit patient population | | | |
| 21. accountability of head nurse | | | |
| 22. mechanisms for interviewing and selecting staff for the unit | | | |
| 23. mechanisms for obtaining admitting orders on patients | | | |
| 24. method of patient care delivery on unit | | | |
| 25. unit medication practices | | | |
| 26. discharge planning mechanisms on unit | | | |
| 27. unit mechanisms to deal with patient valuables and confidentiality of patient information | | | |
| 28. mechanisms for data collection about unit utilization and patient population | | | |
| 29. controlling duration of patient stay on unit | | | |
| 30. responsibilities of attending and consulting physicians using the nursing unit | | | |

The correct responses are:

| TOPICS | ELEMENT (number) | MAIN BODY ( ) | ADDENDUM ( ) |
|---|---|---|---|
| 1. nurses' limitation of practice. | IX | X | |
| 2. relationship of unit with admitting office | VI | X | |
| 3. bed size | I | X | |
| 4. narrative | IV | | X |
| 5. preventing microshock hazards | VII | | X |
| 6. equipment check frequency | VII | | X |
| 7. orientation of unit personnel | VIII | X (summary) | X (detailed) |
| 8. relationship of unit to essential support services | VII | X | X (if very detailed) |
| 9. role of charge nurse | VIII | | X (DOC Method) |
| 10. use of nursing process on unit | VIII | | X (as above) |
| 11. accountability of LPN to RN staff | VIII | | X (as above) |

| TOPICS | ELEMENT (number) | MAIN BODY ( ) | ADDENDUM ( ) |
|---|---|---|---|
| 12. required continuing education activities | VIII | X | |
| 13. crash cart checklist | VII | | X |
| 14. limitations of unit in dealing with patient populations and clinical issues | VI | X | |
| 15. organizational chart for unit | IV | | X |
| 16. replacement of broken equipment | VII | X | |
| 17. infection control issues for unit | VII | X (summary) | X (detailed) |
| 18. staffing patterns for the unit | VIII | | X |
| 19. discharge criteria | VI | X | |
| 20. provision of hemodialysis to unit patient population | VII | X | |
| 21. accountability of head nurse | IV | X | |
| 22. mechanisms for interviewing and selecting staff for the unit | VIII | X | |
| 23. mechanisms for obtaining admitting orders on patients | VI | X | |
| 24. method of patient care delivery on unit | VIII | | X |
| 25. unit medication practices | VII | | X |
| 26. discharge planning mechanisms on unit | VI | X | |
| 27. unit mechanisms to deal with patient valuables and confidentiality of patient information | VII | X | |
| 28. mechanisms for data collection about unit utilization and patient population | III | X (listed) | (collections) X (tool) |
| 29. controlling duration of patient stay on unit | VI | X | |
| 30. responsibilities of attending and consulting physicians using the nursing unit | IV | X | |

# EXERCISE #4: ANALYZING A PROCEDURE

Instructions: Read the following Procedure completely.

Then analyze its strengths and weaknesses using the directions for procedure development in chapter 9. For each weakness make recommendations for improvement. Use the following chart for analysis.

| Procedure Analysis Title: Intravenous Pitocin Drip for Post Partums or Abortion | | |
|---|---|---|
| | **Weaknesses** | |
| **Strengths** | **Problem** | **Suggestions for Improvement** |
| | | |

| Procedure: | INTRAVENOUS PITOCIN DRIP FOR POST PARTUMS OR ABORTION |
|---|---|
| Policy: | All patients on this medication will be in the Labor and Delivery area for proper monitoring and safety factors. |
| General Info: | The purpose of IV pitocin is to stimulate/improve uterine contraction. Additional patient therapeutic objectives include: |

1. To control bleeding in post partum patients.
2. To assist in the expulsion of the fetus or placenta in inevitable abortion.
3. To use in saline abortion if contractions are not present or ineffective after 24 hours.

*NOTE:*

1. Pitocin should not be given simultaneously by more than one route.
2. Pitocin should be used for induction of labor only in Labor and Delivery according to L & D policy.

*EQUIPMENT:*

1. IV pole.
2. IV fluids as prescribed.
3. Pitocin as ordered from pharmacy.
4. Appropriate tubing.
5. IVAC Controller, for greater control of administration.

## PROCEDURE:

1. Prepare equipment.

    a. Check physician's order for correct drug, dosage and route.

    b. Obtain medication/solution from pharmacy or add medication and label.

    c. Obtain IVAC Controller from pharmacy.

2. Prepare patient.

    a. Check for allergies and identify patient by name and identification band.

    b. Explain procedure and expected outcome.

    c. Take and record blood pressure and pulse to establish baseline.

3. Establish patient IV and start drip.

4. In the post-partum patient monitor for expected outcome.

    a. The drip rate should be adjusted as necessary to control bleeding or as ordered by a physician.

## RATIONALE:

Usually 10 to 40 units of Pitocin for 1000cc of solution but may vary according to the patient's needs, clinical situation, and physician's discretion.

1.) Pitocin is usually added to $D_5W$ or 0.9% NaC1. Do not mix with protein containing solutions (i.e. Aminosyn, Freamine.)

2.) If added to IV on the area (when pharmacy closed) use a filter needle (available in pharmacy) to add medication to IV bottle to eliminate minute glass particles from the broken ampule.

Assess emotional status of patient and reassure as necessary.

Use an IVAC controller for greater accuracy in administration.

a. Excess bleeding can be noted to be above one saturated pad per hour.

b. Usual rate for other than excess bleeding is 10 U Pitocin per 1000cc fluid every 6-8 hours.

c. Each physician has his own protocol for excess bleeding (up to 40 U Pitocin in 1000cc fluid can be ordered. The rate of infusion is usually four hours or more.)

b. Monitor and record blood pressure and pulse at least every four hours during drip.

Tachycardia and mild hypotension may occur and are transient.
Always assess patient with hypotension for hemorrhage. Hypertension may occur from fluid overload and from rapid infusion of Pitocin.

c. Monitor and record intake and output during drip.

Pitocin may produce a antidiuretic effect which may lead to fluid retention and fluid overload.

d. Document pertinent observations regarding patient's response, tolerance and results of the drip.

5. In the abortion patient.

a. In the patient with an inevitable abortion the drip rate of Pitocin should be adjusted as necessary to control uterine contractions for expulsion of the fetus as ordered by physician.

1. Pitocin is usually administered at 10 U in 1000cc fluid over 4-6 hours.
2. The rate of Pitocin is adjusted to produce strong enough contractions to stimulate passage of the embryo, but mild enough to be tolerated by the patient. (N.B. Contractions can be felt as to the severity by palpating the firmness of the uterus.)
3. Uterine contractions should be no closer than every two minutes and no longer than 60-80 seconds. (If a tetanic contraction occurs, *slow Pitocin rate immediately.*)

b. In the saline abortion, Pitocin is used to commence labor after 24 hours if saline is ineffective in stimulating labor.

c. Use Pitocin to control contractions and excessive bleeding after the passage of the embryo and placenta.

d. Monitor and record blood pressure and pulse at least every four hours during drip.

e. Monitor and record intake and output during drip.

f. Document pertinent observations regarding patient response, tolerance, and results of the drip in the patient's record.

1000cc fluid with 10 U Pitocin is usually given every 8 hours.

Tachycardia and hypotension may occur at beginning of drip. Hypertension may occur from fluid overload or possibly in patients receiving a vasoconstrictor drug in conjunction with caudal block anesthesia.

Pitocin may produce an antidiuretic effect leading to fluid retention and overload.

Compare your analysis to those listed below.

| | Weaknesses | |
| Strengths | Problem | Suggestions for Improvement |
|---|---|---|
| 1. Appropriate topic for procedure content is mixing and hanging (administering) a titrated drug mixture. | 1. Title not complete with use of word "procedure." | 1. Change title to "Administration of IV Pitocin Procedure". |
| 2. Style adequate with equipment listed and procedural content outlined in 2 columns of "what to do" and "important consideration points." | 2. Do not mix policy with procedure/psychomotor skill. | 2. Eliminate the word "policy". Change to "purpose" and direct this at the nurse. Move original statement to "Supportive Data". |
| 3. Detail adequate and flow of information logical. | 3. General information too long; use of this term often invites excessive content, adding to much length to overall procedure. | 3. Eliminate the term "General Information" and replace with "Supportive Data". Limit this to approximately 2″ of content strictly focusing on:<br>— indications for procedure,<br>— definitions of terms,<br>— circumstances of administration such as who can do.<br>Eliminate "note" as this is redundant. All content is "Supportive Data". |
| | 4. Equipment list single column, wasting space. | 4. Double column equipment list to conserve space. |
| | 5. Left hand column should not duplicate the term "procedure." | 5. Title column "Steps". |
| | 6. Right hand column should not reflect "rationale" as this is also an invitation to insert excessive content. | 6. Title column "Key Points" and limit to content which is absolutely essential for the nurse to safely carry out the procedure—focus on risk management here! |
| | 7. Violates the definition and limitations of a procedure by addressing nursing care. Most of content has nothing to do with administering the drug. | 7. Stop procedure after drug is mixed and hung on the patient. Take remainder of content and place in more appropriate format—protocol. Title would be "Pitocin IV Drip Protocol." Set up in protocol format, organize, and expand content as necessary. |
| | 8. Approval date and mechanism not clear. | 8. Add the word "Approval" along with the date and mechanisms. Follow this with next review date and last revision date. |
| | 9. References absent. | 9. Include one clinical reference. |
| | 10. Distribution absent. | 10. Add "Distribution" to indicate to whom this procedure applies and where it can be found. |

Did you pick up on all the problem areas? Again, if you feel weak in this area or need to brush up, review chapter 9. The information used in this exercise will be useful to evaluate your current procedures and provide a written record of your analysis so that when you begin to rewrite your procedures, you can rank them and tackle those with the most weaknesses first.

## EXERCISE #5: ANALYZING A PROTOCOL

Instructions: Read the following protocol completely, then analyze its strengths and weaknesses using the directions for protocol development in chapter 9. Use the following chart for analysis.

| Protocol Analysis<br>Title: Anticonvulsant Protocol | | |
| --- | --- | --- |
| | Weaknesses | |
| Strengths | Problem | Suggestions for Improvement |
| | | |

## ANTICONVULSANT PROTOCOL

PURPOSE: To specify nursing management of patients on anticonvulsants.

LEVEL: INDEPENDENT

CONTENT:

1. ASSESSMENT: All patients will be assessed each shift for seizure activity.

2. EVALUATION OF EFFECTIVENESS: Effective treatment results in no seizure activity.

3. SIDE EFFECTS: Drowsiness, photophobia, nystagmus, dizziness, restlessness, G.I. disturbances. Most noticeable during initiation of therapy and may be dose related.

4. REPORTING TO MD: Report continued seizure and drug blood levels which are outside of therapeutic range immediately.

5. PATIENT INSTRUCTION: Oral anticonvulsants should not be abruptly withdrawn as this may precipitate seizures or status epilepticus. Patients should be taught to take their medication exactly as prescribed. Since anticonvulsants may cause drowsiness, patients should be counseled to discuss with their doctor activities such as driving and operating machinery.

6. DOCUMENTATION: Assessment parameters will be charted each shift. If an anticonvulsant is being given in the presence of seizure activity, there must

be documentation of continued presence or absence of seizures and action taken. Record patient teaching measures.

7. SPECIAL CARE ISSUES:

   a. Diazepam (Valium IV)—The RN may administer Valium IV push as an anticonvulsant only to a patient on a respirator at a rate of 1 mg/minute or to a patient not on a respirator when a physician is in attendance. When not on a respirator, the patient's respiratory rate must be documented before and every five minutes after administration for 20 minutes unless impossible due to seizure activity.

   b. Phenobarbitol (IV)—May be administered IV push by RN as a single dose, not to exceed 100 mg over five minutes. Respiratory rate and B/P, must be documented before administration and every five minutes for at least 10 minutes or until stable.

   c. Diphenylhydantoin (Dilantin IV)—The RN may administer Dilantin IV push at a rate not to exceed 50 mg/minute. If the patient is not seizing, B/P and pulse must be monitored before and every five minutes after administration for at least 10 minutes or until stable. Use caution in patients with bradycardia and heart block. It should be injected into a plain NS IV, as close to the site as possible. If another IV solution is used, the line must be flushed with 10cc NS before and after Dilantin injection.

   d. IV Ativan—The RN may administer Ativan for continuous seizures as a one time dose of 2 mg IV push over 2 minutes. Dose may be repeated once within 30 minutes. B/P and respiratory rate must be documented before and every five minutes after administration for 20 minutes unless impossible due to seizure activity.

REFERENCE:     PDR, 1985
APPROVAL:      P&T Committee, 10/85
               Nursing Standards Committee, 10/85
               Nursing Management Team, 10/85
REVIEW:        10/85
REVISION:      10/86
DISTRIBUTION: All Nursing Units

Compare your analysis to the following:

| | Weaknesses | |
| Strengths | Problems | Suggestions for Improvement |
| --- | --- | --- |
| 1. Excellent topic for Protocol content in the area of drug management.<br><br>2. Title clear and concise.<br><br>3. Purpose well stated.<br><br>4. Level appropriately stated: content is limited to autonomous nursing function.<br><br>5. Content organized logically in terms of assessment, evaluation, side effects, patient instruction, and documentation.<br><br>6. General nursing management content appropriately placed at the beginning of the protocol.<br><br>7. Specific nursing actions for each drug delineated under "Special Concerns".<br><br>8. Content directed at top four drugs: useful priority setting.<br><br>9. Approval dates, mechanisms, review, and revision dates, and distribution clear. | 1. Content of nursing care lacks specificity. Content is often stated as information (i.e., listing of side effects) instead of spelling out nursing directives.<br><br>2. Failure of nursing care content to begin with "action verbs" directing staff to perform clear and measurable nursing actions.<br><br><br><br>3. Lack of numbered (1, 2, 3, and so forth) nursing actions. Paragraph style statements take too long to read and also fail to set care priorities. | 1. List words like assessment, side effects, evaluation of effectiveness, patient instruction, documentation, and so forth as "Key Words" in the left margin and organize care statements around these.<br><br>2. Add specificity to nursing care measures. Eliminate information giving, and start each nursing care statement with an action verb such as:<br>— assess, observe . . .<br>— report . . .<br>— document . . .<br>— counsel patients . . .<br>— validate . . .<br>— administer . . .<br>Focus not only on the specificity of content, but also on the sophistication of the nursing management.<br><br>3. Number nursing care actions in priority of care to be given. |

NOTE: In consideration of this challenging activity, an extra protocol entitled "Anticonvulsant Protocol" is included to allow you to compare and contrast a weak protocol with a strong one, following the Model's approach to protocol development yet staying within the alloted length of two pages (back/front).

# HOSPITAL
# DEPARTMENT OF NURSING

*ANTICONVULSANT PROTOCOL (Using the Marker Model)*

*PURPOSE:* To specify nursing responsibilities in the management of patients on anticonvulsants (phenobarbital, valium, ativan, dilantin).

*LEVEL:* Independent (requires nursing order only after drug initiated by physician).

*SUPPORTIVE DATA:* Antiseizure medications may be grouped as anticonvulsants (dilantin) or as barbituates (phenobarbital) or anxiety reducing hyponotics (valium, antivan). The drugs of choice or combination are dependent on the type of seizure activity and its history. Most of the drugs have dose related side effects making nursing assessment and patient education important to safe therapy.

CONTENT:

SEIZURE
ASSESSMENT

1. Assess patient *each shift* for presence of seizure activity including grand mal, twitching, numbness, or momentary lapses in alertness; record P/A in shift summary in NPR.

NEUROLOGIC
ASSESSMENT

2. Perform neurological vital signs a *minimum of once each shift* and record on neuro FS/VS sheet including:

   - motion/strength/coordination in all extremities,
   - pupillary response/size including P/A of abnormal, pupil reactions such as nystagmus and diplopia,
   - B/P, A/R rate, respirations for one minute.

ASSESSMENT FOR
SIDE EFFECTS

3. Observe for common side effects of this drug category each shift; if patient alert, instruct patient/SO to report same to staff. Include:

   - excessive drowsiness/dizziness,
   - photophobia,
   - nausea/vomiting/anorexia/constipation,
   - ataxia.

   NOTE   Since drugs in this category are metabolized by the liver and excreted by the kidney, *be alert to toxic accumulation* in patients with liver/renal dysfunction.

SAFETY/
CORRECTIVE
ACTION

4. Maintain plastic airway and suction devices at bedside as specified in "Seizure Protocol".

5. *If drowsiness/dizziness/ataxia is excessive problem:*

   a. Keep patient in bed with side rails up and low position.

   b. Use chair with posey and keep call light within reach.

   c. Ambulate with assistance only.

   d. Record B/P *twice per shift* to observe for excessive hypotension.

   e. Assist with all meals and physical care (due to ataxia).

   f. Do not allow patient to smoke unattended.

6. *If photophobia present:*

   a. Keep drapes/blinds drawn.

   b. Use room nightlight—not overheads.

   c. Keep pupil check to a minimum in duration to reduce pain.

   d. Direct patient to wear sun glasses.

7. *If GI symptoms present:*

   a. Maintain on clear liquids if N/V present.

   b. Obtain dietary consult for anorexia.

   c. Force fluids to minimum of 1500 cc/day; monitor daily BM's; discuss use of laxatives and stool softeners with physician.

8. Discuss all side effects with physician; may be dose related; may decrease with time or dose modifications; reassure patient that some dose adjustment is usually necessary.

*EVALUATION OF EFFECT/ COMMUNICATION WITH MD*

9. In *shift assessment,* note the following in Nursing Progress Record:

   a. Time period since last seizure activity, time between seizure episodes, and reduced intensity or frequency of activity.

   b. P/A side effects and reduction with time or dose change.

   c. Discuss with physician lab blood level determinations; keep physician informed daily (day shift) as to lab values and patient response in 9(a), 9 (b); chart all discussions with physician.

*PATIENT EDUCATION*

10. Inform patient during hospitalization therapy, the name of his drug/s:

   a. Have him repeat each and its purpose.

   b. Have him open unit dose packet and observe him take PO meds.

   c. Establish at each administration the patient's perception of side effects presence.

   d. If patient to be discharged on drug/s, review the following. Obtain repeat explanation by patient/SO.

| CONTENT | DATE | RN | UNDERSTOOD |
|---|---|---|---|
| 1. Take medications q̄ day without interruption. | | | |
| 2. Danger of arbitrarily discontinuing/ skipping drug. | | | |
| 3. Name of drugs written on paper with purpose. | | | |
| 4. Side effects of drugs, including: <br>— drowsiness, <br>— GI symptoms, <br>— dizziness, <br>— photophobia. | | | |
| 5. Dangers to avoid: <br>— use of drugs/ETOH <br>— driving/using machinery | | | |
| 6. To see MD when told, if seizures continue, S.E. | | | |

*DOCUMENTATION*  11. Document as specified all assessment, corrective actions, side effects, physician communication on NFS and NPR.

12. Record that *Anticonvulsant Protocol* has been implemented each shift on the Standards Flowsheet (per guidelines).

13. Record patient education if discharged on medications as tool specifies.

*DOCUMENTATION DURING ACUTE SEIZURE ACTIVITY*  14. If drug given during seizure activity:

a. Record special note in NPR indicating seizure type, character, time, post ictal condition, and medications given (dose, concentration, route, patient response).

b. Record follow up assessment 10, 20, 30, 60 minutes later to evaluate effectiveness of drug.

*SPECIAL CONCERNS*  15. PHENOBARB (IV)

a. May be given IVP by RN as single dose not to exceed *120 mg over 5 minutes.*

b. Record respiratory rate, B/P, HR before and q̄ 5 minutes × 15 and q̄ hour × 2 to assess for respiratory depression.

c. Implement proper positioning of airway and pulmonary toilette to prevent obstruction/atelectasis from lethargy.

d. Maintain safety precautions (previously identified).

16. DILANTIN (phenytoin) (IV)

a. May be given IVP by RN at rate *not to exceed 50 mg/min;* line must be flushed with 10cc NS prior to and after single doses.

b. Record apical HR and B/P before and *q̄ 5 minutes × 15 and q̄ hour × 2* to assess for cardiovascular depression.

c. If continuous drip started:
   • dilute in saline/flush line with NS;
   • piggyback to 250cc NS;
   • use controller;
   • assess patient/infusion q̄ hour for:
     — correction infusion rate,
     — evaluation of seizures,
     — apical HR and B/P.

d. Observe all patients on Dilantin (PO/IM/IV) for HR < 55 or > 110.

e. Review old EKG's and do not administer if HR < 55 or heartblock present.

f. Report negative side effects on V/S to MD and slow/hold drug.

g. Note that maximum effect not achieved for 7-10 days with level of 10-20 mcg/ml—observe for seizure activity during that time.

h. DO NOT WITHDRAW DRUG ABRUPTLY—status epilepticus may ensue.

i. ADMINISTER (PO) WITH MEALS TO ↓ GI SYMPTOMS.

j. Discuss with MD, CBC/platelet count values determination to check for possible hemopoietic complications.

k. OBSERVE FOR SKIN RASH q̄ DAY (instruct patient to report this).

l. OBSERVE GUMS q̄ WEEK for hyperplasia; give mouth care (or encourage patient's self care) with brushing and message to discourage tissue buildup; OBSERVE FOR BLEEDING GUMS (instruct patient).

17. VALIUM (diazepam) (IV)

    a. May be given IVP by RN at rate of *1mg/min ONLY TO PATIENTS ON RESPIRATORS* or to patients not on ventilatory support *IN THE PRESENCE OF A PHYSICIAN.*

    b. Record apical HR, B/P, respiratory rate and quality *before and q̄ 5 minutes × 15 and q̄ hour × 2* to assess for respiratory depression and hypotension.

    c. Maintain airway and pulmonary pro-phylaxis, including *T, C, DB q̄ 2 hours.*

    d. Have suction, oral airways, and resus. bag at bedside.

    e. DO NOT ADMINISTER TO PATIENTS WITH ACUTE NARROW ANGLE GLAUCOMA.

    f. Observe IV site for phlebitis, thrombosis, local irritation each shift; rotate IV infusion sites *q̄ 48 hours;* avoid small veins—use brachial for direct IV push.

    g. Normally valium is not diluted; if physician insists, mix in concentration of 50mg/1000cc NS with filter.

    h. Institute all safety measures to prevent self injury.

    i. Discuss use of minimum doses with MD when patient already on narcotics, pheno-thiazines, MAO inhibitors, anti-depressants.

18. ATIVAN IV

    a. RN's may administer this drug IVP for con-tinuous seizures as a *one time dose of 2 mg IVP over 2 minutes;* must be diluted in an equal volume; aspirate frequently to prevent extravasation; dose may be *repeated × 1 within 30 minutes.*

    b. Observe for respiratory depression and have respiratory support equipment on standby.

c. Record apical HR, B/P, respiratory rate and quality *before and q̄ 5 minutes × 15 and q̄ hour × 2* to assess for respiratory depression.

d. Observe for extreme drowsiness and implement safety precautions.

REFERENCE: PDR, 1985
APPROVAL: P&T Committee, 10/85
Nursing Standards Committee, 10/85
Nursing Management Team, 10/85
REVIEW: 10/85
REVISION: 10/86
DISTRIBUTION: All Nursing Units

Review the information in Chapter 9 if you had any difficulty with this exercise. As with Exercise 4, this information provides documentation of current status and a barometer to monitor progress in writing protocols.

## EXERCISE #6: PROCESS MATCHING

Instructions: Read through the 24 Process issues listed below and determine which of the six formats is most appropriate for that issue. In some cases more than one format may be appropriate. Place a check in the appropriate format box and compare your answers with those on page 6.

| ISSUE | JOB DESCRIPTION | PERFORMANCE STANDARDS | PROCEDURE | PROTOCOL | GUIDELINES | STANDARD OF CARE |
|---|---|---|---|---|---|---|
| 1. I/O Record | | | | | | |
| 2. AIDS | | | | | | |
| 3. ventilator care | | | | | | |
| 4. Immuno-suppressed patient | | | | | | |
| 5. diabetes | | | | | | |
| 6. hypoglycemia | | | | | | |
| 7. nursing data base | | | | | | |
| 8. starting/discontinuing an IV | | | | | | |
| 9. care planning | | | | | | |
| 10. hemodialysis | | | | | | |
| 11. anaphyactic shock | | | | | | |
| 12. post resuscitation care | | | | | | |
| 13. assisting with bedside bronchoscopy | | | | | | |
| 14. ABGs (drawing) | | | | | | |
| 15. hip fracture | | | | | | |
| 16. crutchfield tongs | | | | | | |
| 17. issues of patient care emergency that staff must be able to manage in day to day unit function | | | | | | |
| 18. chemotherapy | | | | | | |
| 19. hyperbilirubinemia | | | | | | |
| 20. MI | | | | | | |
| 21. barbiturate OD | | | | | | |
| 22. infant bonding | | | | | | |
| 23. suicide | | | | | | |
| 24. use of nursing diagnosis | | | | | | |

The correct answers are:

| ISSUE | JOB DESCRIPTION | PERFORMANCE STANDARDS | PROCEDURE | PROTOCOL | GUIDELINES | STANDARD OF CARE |
|---|---|---|---|---|---|---|
| 1. I/O Record | | | | X | | |
| 2. AIDS | | | | | | X |
| 3. ventilator care | | | X | | | |
| 4. Immuno-suppressed patient | | | X | | | |
| 5. diabetes | | | | | | X |
| 6. hypoglycemia | | | X | | | |
| 7. nursing data base | | | | X | | |
| 8. starting/discontinuing an IV | | | X | | | |
| 9. care planning | X | X | | | | |
| 10. hemodialysis | | | X | X | | |
| 11. anaphyactic shock | | | X | | | |
| 12. post resuscitation care | | | X | | | |
| 13. assisting with bedside bronchoscopy | | | X | | | |
| 14. ABGs (drawing) | | | X | | | |
| 15. hip fracture | | | | | | X |
| 16. crutchfield tongs | | | X | X | | |
| 17. issues of patient care emergency that staff must be able to manage in day to day unit function | X | X | | | | |
| 18. chemotherapy | | | X | X | | |
| 19. hyperbilirubinemia | | | X | | | |
| 20. MI | | | | | | X |
| 21. barbiturate OD | | | | | | X |
| 22. infant bonding | | | X | | | |
| 23. suicide | | | X | | | |
| 24. use of nursing diagnosis | X | X | | | | |

If you had difficulty with this exercise, review the content in Unit III.

## EXERCISE #7: INTEGRATING PROTOCOLS AND STANDARDS OF CARE

Instructions: Read the list of standards of care in column A and select the priority protocols from column B most likely to be used to support each standard of care. Place the letter of the protocols in the parentheses beside the standard of care.

COLUMN A (Standard of Care)

1. MI
   (   ) (   ) (   )
2. Aortic Femoral Bypass
   (   ) (   )
3. CHF
   (   ) (   )
4. Laryngectomy
   (   ) (   )
5. GI Bleeding
   (   ) (   ) (   )
6. Colon resection with fistula complication
   (   ) (   ) (   )
7. AIDS
   (   ) (   )
8. Laminectomy
   (   ) (   )
9. Epiglottitis
   (   )
10. TAH (28 yr old woman)
    (   ) (   )
11. Acute Leukemia
    (   ) (   ) (   ) (   )
12. Spinal Cord Transection (parapalegic)
    (   ) (   )
13. Hemigastrectomy
    (   ) (   )

COLUMN B (Protocols)

a. Chest Pain Management
b. Depression/Grieving
c. Immobility
d. Alteration in Skin Integrity
e. Supplemental $0_2$ Management
f. Artificial Airway Management
g. Immuno Suppression Management
h. GU Intubation
i. GI Intubation
j. Shock (Hypovalemic)
k. DV Therapy
l. Anticoagulant
m. Post-op
n. Chronic Pain Management
o. Complicated Wound Management
p. Arrhythmia Management
q. Vasodilator Therapy Management
r. Blood Products Administration Management

The answers to Exercise 7 are:

COLUMN A (Standard of Care)

1. MI (a) (p) (k)
2. Aortic Femoral Bypass (m) (k)
3. CHF (q) (e)
4. Laryngectomy (m) (f)
5. GI Bleeding (j) (k) (r)
6. Colon resection with fistula complication (m) (o) (k)
7. AIDS (g) (b)
8. Laminectomy (c) (m)
9. Epiglottitis (e)
10. TAH (28 yr old woman) (m) (b)
11. Acute Leukemia (b) (d) (g) (n)
12. Spinal Cord Transection (parapalegic) (d) (h)
13. Hemigastrectomy (m) (i)

COLUMN B (Protocols)

a. Chest Pain Management
b. Depression/Grieving
c. Immobility
d. Alteration in Skin Integrity
e. Supplemental $O_2$ Management
f. Artificial Airway Management
g. Immuno Suppression Management
h. GU Intubation
i. GI Intubation
j. Shock (Hypovalemic)
k. DV Therapy
l. Anticoagulant
m. Post-op
n. Chronic Pain Management
o. Complicated Wound Management
p. Arrhythmia Management
q. Vasodilator Therapy Management
r. Blood Products Administration Management

Having completed all the exercises in this chapter, you have confirmed your understanding of the Marker Model and your ability to put it into practice. You're now ready to begin planning and implementing nursing standards.

# Chapter 13:   Creating the Standards Manual

## CRITICAL ISSUES

In setting up your Standards Manuals, keep four critical points in mind.

First, the term *Policy/Procedure* is outmoded and inadequate to define our nursing practice and the traditional Policy/Procedure Manual too rigid to house your new standards. There is no logical way to locate performance standards, protocols, guidelines, and standards of care under the limited category of "Policy/Procedure". So call the Manual what it really is—*Standards Manual.*

Second, separate GENERIC STANDARDS and UNIT SPECIFIC STANDARDS. Generic standards are those that apply to all staff and patients and are applicable to any nursing unit. Specific standards are those that are applicable to a particular unit or limited group of units. This separation helps control the size of the standards manual and prevents staff intimidation due to excessive volume of a single manual. All of our work has been divided into "generic" and "specific". There is **generic structure** (Policy) for the Department of Nursing and **unit specific structure** for each nursing unit. There are the generic **job descriptions** and the **unit based performance standards**; there are **procedures, protocols,** and **forms with guidelines** used housewide that are generic and those that are limited to use in selected areas that are unit specific. Thus each nursing area would have two standards manuals:

- DEPARTMENT OF NURSING GENERIC STANDARDS MANUAL
- UNIT SPECIFIC NURSING STANDARDS MANUAL

Third, each standards manual has two sections set up according to the Marker Model. The front section is structure and houses the policies for the Department of Nursing or Nursing Unit. The policies are written as a set in an outline, paragraph style covering the 13 elements of structure for the department or the 9 elements for the unit. The structure standards come first because they are the foundation of your system, the basis for your decision making, and foundation for your process function. The back section is devoted to process standards. These make up the bulk of your manual and contain the process formats in the order of their development and sophistication—job descriptions, performance standards, procedures, protocols, forms/guidelines, standards of care. Below is the suggested set up of both manuals:

## DEPARTMENT OF NURSING GENERIC STANDARDS MANUAL

*TITLE:* Hospital/Facility
Department of Nursing
Generic Nursing Standards Manual

*First Major Tab:* STRUCTURE STANDARDS
(POLICIES covering 13 elements of structure)

    I. Department Description
    II. Purpose of Department
    III. Philosophy of Department
    IV. Objectives of Department
    V. Administration/Organization
    VI. Hours of Operation
    VII. Use of Nursing Areas
    VIII. Use of Staff and Staffing Practices
    IX. Maintenance of Professional Practice System
    X. Governing Rules
    XI. Selection/Retention/Orientation/Education/Development/Evaluation/Credentialing of Nursing Personnel
    XII. Nursing Quality Assurance Program
    XIII. Nursing Responsibilities (general)

Second Major Tab: PROCESS STANDARDS
    *Format Tab:* JOB DESCRIPTIONS/CAREER LADDERS/EVALUATION TOOLS
    *Format Tab:* GENERIC PROCEDURES (alphabetized)
    *Format Tab:* GENERIC PROTOCOLS (alphabetized)
    *Format Tab:* GENERIC FORMS/GUIDELINES (alphabetized)
    *Format Tab:* STANDARDS OF CARE (No actual Care Plans—only a brief discussion of how they are used and can be found in the Unit Manuals. Also include a list by clinical area of standards of care that currently exist.)

Note that in addition to the main body of Department of Nursing policies covering content in the 13 elements would be the detailed addenda under each element. Each addendum would be tabbed, titled, and alphabetized and arranged after the set of structure standards, following the organizational chart and narrative. Also note that this manual contains no actual standards of care.

# UNIT SPECIFIC NURSING STANDARDS MANUAL

*TITLE:* Hospital Facility
Department of Nursing
_____ Unit Nursing Standards Manual

*First Major Tab:*     STRUCTURE STANDARDS
                       (POLICIES covering 9 elements of structure)

    I. Unit Description
    II. Purpose of Unit
    III. Objectives of Unit
    IV. Administration/Organization of Unit
    V. Hours of Operation
    VI. Use of Nursing Unit
    VII. Governing Rules
    VIII. Staffing
    IX. Nursing Responsibilities (specific)

Second Major Tab: PROCESS STANDARDS
   *Format Tab:* PERFORMANCE STANDARDS
   *Format Tab:* PROCEDURES (alphabetized)
   *Format Tab:* PROTOCOLS (alphabetized)
   *Format Tab:* FORMS/GUIDELINES (alphabetized)
   *Format Tab:* STANDARDS OF CARE (alphabetized)

Note that in addition to the main body of unit level policies covering content in the 9 elements would be the specific addenda under each element. Each addendum would be tabbed, titled, and alphabetized and arranged after the set of structure standards, following the organizational chart and narrative. Unlike the Department Standards Generic Manual, the standards of care for the major patient populations admitted to the area are located here.

Fourth, color coding of the manuals by some predesignated method will enhance the staff's ability to identify critically important manuals in the area. While staff must be generally familiar with many reference books on their unit, i.e., lab, dietary, personnel, etc., their main manuals are those of the Department of Nursing and their specific units. Color coding the Department of Nursing Manual makes this uniform throughout the department while making it stand apart from the rest of the references. Color coding by division or cluster of units, i.e. red for Critical Care, blue for Medical/Surgical, yellow for Maternal-Child Health, purple for Psychiatry, clearly locates the specific unit standards.

When these two manuals stand side by side, they not only define professional practice, but serve as a basis for two more manuals—the Unit Based Orientation Manual and the Unit Based Quality Assurance Manual. These two important aspects of unit activity and managerial function are logical extensions of the standards development project.

# ADDITIONAL CONSIDERATIONS

The set up of the standards manual just presented demands some reconsideration of common approaches used in traditional policy/procedure manuals. One reconsideration is page numbering. In a standards manual, the pages are not numbered consecutively from beginning to end. Only each standard is numbered according to its content pages. This is because each part of the manual will probably grow at different rates. The structure section and performance standards section of process should be completed within about six to eight months. But the remainder of the process section will continue to grow for probably over a year. Also, new issues will always emerge which will need to be added to the manual. Numbering pages is too rigid to allow the content to rapidly expand. For example, if you develop a set of structure standards that is fifteen pages long, you would number the pages consecutively one to fifteen. Each supportive addendum is then tabbed, given an alphabetical reference in the set of policies, and organized behind the main body of policies. If you had addenda A - T, each addendum would have individually numbered pages. This allows organized alphabetized expansion and the addition or deletion of addenda as needed without concern for adjusting the page numbering system. Another example would be protocols. If you wrote a protocol on "Immobility" located under "I" of the process-protocol section and then developed another protocol on "Hyperalimentation" at a later date, the new protocol is simply inserted under "H" in the process-protocol section without regard for consecutive numbering. So number the pages of individual standards, but do not number all pages consecutively from beginning to end.

Another reconsideration is indexing the manual. Traditionally, there is one master index, alphabetically laid out, extensive in length, and often cross indexed by multiple subjects. There is no such index to the standards manual. Instead there is a brief overview and introduction to the manual for staff to get an idea of how the generic and unit specific manuals are organized. Then each section is indexed simply by listing the content to be found there. The list will be alphabetized but limited to the standards in that section, i.e., procedures, protocols, standards of care.

This system of organizing standards can be learned by all those who have to use it because it is a SYSTEM. If a staff member is oriented properly to the Marker Model, its approach, methodology, and terminology and introduced to the manuals early in his/her employment, then location of reference items is quick and easy.

# ST. HOSPITAL'S HOSPITAL
## DEPARTMENT OF NURSING
## 8 WEST UNIT
## NURSING STANDARDS
## MANUAL

# INTRODUCTION/OVERVIEW OF NURSING STANDARDS MANUAL

## TO ALL MEMBERS OF THE NURSING STAFF

As part of the philosophy of the Department of Nursing and in meeting professional and regulatory requirements, the Department has written nursing standards to define systems function, staff performance, and patient care. We have adopted the *Marker Model, Hierarchy of Nursing Standards* as our framework for defining professional nursing practice. This overview will introduce you to the standards manuals and explain their use.

In lieu of a traditional policy and procedure manual, we maintain two standards manuals on each nursing unit. While they contain both policy and procedure, they are called standards manuals because they contain more standards that comprehensively define nursing in our system. You are expected to familiarize yourself with these references and use them actively in your practice. All standards are divided into **GENERIC** and **SPECIFIC**. The **GENERIC MANUAL** is on each nursing unit and contains information about general nursing practice. In addition, each nursing unit has its own **UNIT SPECIFIC MANUAL**. There is no duplication of content, only separation of information to reduce the volume of each manual and make it easier for you to use.

The green manual is the **Department of Nursing Generic Standards Manual** and contains the policies of the Department of Nursing as **STRUCTURE**. Any issue which concerns the operation of the department as a whole will be found in this set of policies. By reading the outline at the beginning of the structure section, you will become aware of the content addressed here. The second section is **PROCESS** and organizes general nursing practice into six formats. Here you'll find all Department employee **Job Descriptions/Career Ladders/Performance Appraisal** Tools; generic **Procedures, Protocols, Forms** and **Guidelines**; and an explanation of **Standards of Care** use in the system. Each format section has an index to help you locate items. You are expected to study the manual during orientation and be familiar with our terminology and location of items. Any nursing care activities that are similar throughout the nursing areas are defined here.

The blue manual is your **Unit Specific Nursing Standards Manual** for this Medical/Surgical Unit. It contains the policies for the operation of 8 West as **Structure** standards. The content outline preceding the policies shows the topics addressed. Simply scan the outline and refer to the set of policies to locate your concern. The unit policies will refer to a specific structure addendum if one exists for more detail. Please familiarize yourself with the addendum tabs as each addendum is clearly labeled. Finally, the last section of the unit manual is **Process** and is similarly divided by tabs into six **process formats**. This content is very specific to the expectations of staff on 8 West, the patient populations and patient care on the nursing unit.

If what you are looking for is applicable to the entire house, look in the green manual; if it is specific to 8 West, look in the blue manual.

## INDEX TO UNIT STRUCTURE

## GENERAL POLICIES*

I. **DESCRIPTION:** 8 West is a 40 bed medical/surgical unit located on the 8th floor of the Main building. It consists of 16 semiprivate rooms, and 8 private rooms set up for all types of isolation.

II. **PURPOSE:** To provide quality care to adult medical/surgical patients who are acutely ill or injured and in varying stages of recuperation from diagnostic, therapeutic, or surgical interventions.

III. **OBJECTIVES:**

A. To provide an environment conducive to healing through the prompt detection of emergency conditions and through the prevention of complications associated with diseases and disorders; for those patients whose conditions cannot be treated, to provide an environment conducive to death with dignity.

B. To provide the equipment necessary to control pain, promote patient comfort, and to perform required diagnostic and therapeutic procedures.

C. To provide the highest level of nursing and medical management using a collaborative multidisciplinary approach, minimizing the negative physical and psychological effects of disease processes through patient/family education, ultimately restoring the patient to self care.

D. To collect data on all patients admitted to the unit for the purpose of assessing the unit's function. Parameters include:
1. patient's name, age, and diagnoses (primary and secondary);
2. method of admission (direct, emergency, routine, transfer);
3. disposition (home, ECF, hospital, morgue);
4. length of stay;
5. complications (none, infection, code, other).

IV. **ADMINISTRATION AND ORGANIZATION OF UNIT:**

A. 8 West is a general medical-surgical unit organized as a nursing unit within the Department of Nursing. Overall management of the unit is the responsibility of the Patient Care

* Due to the page size of this manual, the 15 page limit was not adhered to.

Supervisor (PCS) with supervision, direction, and support by the Assistant Director of Nursing (ADN), Medical-Surgical areas. Collaboration with physicians and appropriate department heads takes place periodically through formal and informal meetings. See Department of Nursing organization chart and 8 West organization chart for a diagram of these relationships. This will be reviewed annually and updated as necessary to reflect the current organizational relationships in the area.

B. A narrative exists to describe and explain the 8 West organizational chart. It will be maintained concurrently as the organizational chart is revised.

C. Direction of the 8 West nursing unit.

1. Nursing Direction:

   a. The 8 West Patient Care Supervisor (PCS) is an RN with requisite clinical and managerial experience. She is specially selected by the Nursing Administration to assume responsibility for the effective organization and management of 8 West area. He/she has 24 hour responsibility for the effective functioning of the staff including their development and evaluation; the efficient functioning of the 8 West subsystem; and the quality of patient care provided in the setting.

   b. The 8 West PCS assigns a shift coordinator each shift to oversee the 8 (10 or 12) hour shift for the purpose of facilitating unit communications, coordination, and delivery of patient care.

   c. The Nursing Office Supervisor (NOS) is a member of the Nursing Management Team and acts as a resource person to the Shift Coordinator (in the absence of the PCS) providing direction and support during weekend, holidays, and alternate shifts. During her eight hour shifts of duty, she also is responsible for upholding the standards and managing the projects of the PCS and the unit. The NOS contributes to staff development and evaluation of the nursing staff and communicates with the unit PCS on a regular basis regarding staff performance and any problems concerning unit operation or patient care.

   d. The PCS reports to the Assistant Director of Nursing (ADN) of Medical Surgical Areas. While this is a direct line relationship, the PCS maintains authority in managing her unit. The ADN provides direction, support and guidance to the PCS and aids in her development both clinically and administratively. The ADN provides an additional level of clinical expertise and functions as resource to the staff as well as PCS. The ADN is active in periodic supervision, standards development, and quality assurance. She is responsible primarily for development of the division as a subsystem for the Department of Nursing and links the divisional unit with the executive level of the Department of Nursing.

e. The Executive Director of Nursing (DON) is ultimately responsible for the quality of personnel performance and patient care delivered within the Department of Nursing. She meets these responsibilities indirectly through delegation to the qualified Nursing Management Team. The DON links the Department of Nursing with the medical and administrative hierarchy. She is ultimately responsible for the growth of the Nursing Service as a whole in seeing that it responds to the needs of the institution specifically and the Community in general.

2. Medical Direction:

a. The responsibility for directing medical care on 8 West is that of the attending (admitting) physician and associates. This responsibility may be delegated, but only as specified in the Medical Staff Bylaws, through a written order for transfer of services or by consultation.

b. Specific responsibilities of the attending physician on 8 West include:

(1) Completing a history and physical examination on all patients within 48 hours post admission, and documenting the findings in the patients' charts.

(2) Giving clear orders on the medical care plans for all new patients, either in writing or orally with the nursing staff.

(3) Visiting patients daily and updating progress notes to keep the nursing staff informed of changes in medical care plans.

(4) Collaborating daily (on unit or by phone) with the nursing staff in regard to the medical care plan, prognosis, and anticipated discharge.

(5) Complying with the average length of stay for patients coming under the DRG system; alerting the PCS to extended lengths of stay.

(6) Being available to the nursing staff for questions and reports on patients' conditions.

(7) Being present on the unit to see patients when the nursing staff feels that patient condition warrants further medical examination.

(8) Helping to write, approve, and implement standards of care for patients on 8 West.

(9) Contacting consultants and assuming responsibility for clarifying any conflicts that may arise between medical orders, including updating physicians who may be covering patient care.

(10) Meeting regularly with the patient's family/significant others to keep them informed of his medical progress.

(11) Participating in nursing staff development and care conferences.

(12) Assisting in monitoring compliance with Quality Assurance activities on the unit.

c. The Chiefs of the Medical, Surgical, and Special Services will be available to the PCS, shift coordinators, NOS, and ADN to provide medical direction when the attending physician is not available. Chiefs of Service will serve on a liaison committee that meets periodically to discuss management of the unit and the quality of patient care.

d. The responsibilities of the Consulting Physician on 8 West include:

(1) Communicating with the nursing staff to clarify patient care responsibilities so that effective interaction between consultants and the nursing staff can be maintained. This includes specifying when consultant relationships have been terminated.

(2) Charting consultation notes within 24 hours after seeing patients, updating consultant progress notes daily.

(3) Discussing medical care plans with the attending physician to prevent conflicts in medical orders and in the direction of the nursing staff.

(4) Meeting regularly with the patient's family/significant others.

3. Committee Structure:

a. The Medical-Surgical Nurse Physician Liaison committee is an ad hoc group of selected members of the nursing management team and medical staff who meet to:

(1) Build working relationships of trust and respect;

(2) Collaborate on patient care and unit or division issues;

(3) Write and approve standards for patient care;

(4) Facilitate quality assurance activities.

b. The members of this committee will be:

(1) Head nurses of the medical-surgical units, their assistants, and middle managers;

(2) Clinical specialists or instructors;

(3) Departments, as invited to discuss pertinent issues;

(4) The chiefs of medicine, surgery, orthopaedics, and oncology, and other members of the medical staff, as invited to discuss pertinent issues;

(5) Hospital administration representative.

c. The committee will be co-chaired by the Chief of Medicine and the Assistant Director of Medical/Surgical Nursing areas. The agenda will be drawn up one week before each meeting. The group will meet every other month at a designated time. Minutes will be taken and copies sent to the Director of Nursing and the Medical Executive Committee.

d. In addition, professional staff will be selected by appropriate committee chairpersons to participate on committees at the Department of Nursing level and Hospital/Medical Staff level. These RN's will represent the nursing department and unit and assist with committee objectives and communication of activities.

e. 8 West will hold periodic care conferences, approximately two per week, and monthly staff meetings to facilitate patient care and effective staff communication.

V. **HOURS OF OPERATION:** 8 West is a bedded unit providing set hours of care to an average daily census 24 hours a day. Staffing will be adjusted for census changes and increased or decreased acuity levels among the patients on the unit.

VI. **UTILIZATION OF THE UNIT:**

A. Admission Policies

1. All members of the medical staff with active admitting privileges may admit patients to 8 West. Doctors with courtesy privileges must be approved by the Chief of Service. They must request appropriate consultation as

directed by the Chief of Service and as specified by the medical staff bylaws.

2. Patients may be admitted to 8 West in any of the following ways:

   a. *Direct Admissions* are admitted directly from their doctor's offices or their homes, with arrangements made by phone through the admissions office. These patients may transport themselves to the hospital, or they may arrive on the unit with medical orders. These orders may be written by the patient's doctor and brought to the unit by the patient himself, or they may be written in the emergency room after an initial medical assessment there. Medical orders relayed by telephone before the patient's arrival on the unit will also be acceptable for admission.

   b. *Emergency Admissions* are patients admitted from the emergency room. These patients must also arrive on the unit with medical orders, written in by the emergency room physician or relayed by telephone to the unit by the Attending Physician.

   c. *Transfer patients* are admitted to 8 West from other units, such as the intensive care unit, the coronary care unit, or the operating room. The unit transferring the patient will obtain updated medical orders before the transfer and see they accompany the patient to the unit.

   d. *Routine admissions* are patients scheduled in advance for admission to 8 West. These patients may be brought to the unit by admitting clerks or volunteer workers with written medical orders. The admitting officer will obtain these orders or alert the nursing staff on the unit if orders have not been written so the attending physician can be contacted. Physicians are strongly encouraged to send routine admissions with prewritten admission orders.

   e. *Boarders* are patients that because of their particular pathology will benefit from being on a specific unit but due to bed limitations are "temporarily" placed on 8 West. The Admitting Office will identify these patients and collaborate with the 8 West nursing staff to move them as soon as possible. Nursing consultation will be sought with specific unit as appropriate. The Clinical Specialist will be alerted to these patients.

3. Circumstances of Admission:

    a. No patients will be admitted to 8 West unless they arrive with medical orders that specify:

        (1) admitting diagnosis and order to admit to unit;

        (2) code status or directions for the management of a life-threatening crisis;

        (3) diet;

        (4) activity level;

        (5) vital signs and how often they should be taken;

        (6) laboratory tests that need to be scheduled;

        (7) routine medications, especially those the patient takes on his own;

        (8) PRN medications, such as analgesics, laxatives, antacids, and so forth.

    b. Doctors will visit all emergency patients as soon as possible after their admission to 8 West. The RN assigned to the patient will notify the attending physician of the patient's arrival on the unit and of the patient's status.

    c. Doctors will visit all patients on the unit daily and provide appropriate medical documentation on their conditions. All medical responsibilities previously outlined apply.

    d. The admitting officer will inform the nursing staff on the unit as to the sex and smoking status of each patient. There will be no age or race discrimination in the assignment of patients to rooms on the unit. However, the nursing staff will consider a patient's sex, age, acuity level, and smoking status in placing him on the unit. Special arrangements may be made according to hospital policy so that immediate family members of the opposite sex may be placed in the same room.

    e. Nursing responsibilities with regard to the newly admitted patient include:

        (1) Compiling an admission data base by RN's. While non-professional staff members admit a patient, only an RN can complete this initial admission assessment;

        (2) Writing an admission note, also a responsibility of the admitting RN;

    (3)  Acknowledging medical admission orders, also a responsibility of the admitting RN;

    (4)  Developing a care plan as outlined in the unit's policy on delivery of care in addendum J;

    (5)  Entering patient's name to the 8 West patient log, or delegating this to the unit clerk.

4. Criteria for Admission:

  a. Generally, a patient is considered a candidate for admission to 8 West if he is an adult experiencing an acute or potentially acute illness or injury, or an exacerbation of a chronic condition, affecting one or more body system.

  b. Common candidates for admission include:

    (1)  Post-ICU transfer patients from both medical and surgical units;

    (2)  Patients with diseases or disorders requiring diagnostic or therapeutic intervention, such as diabetes mellitus, gastro-intestinal bleeding, abdominal pain, chronic obstructive pulmonary disease, and congestive heart failure;

    (3)  Post-op general anesthesia and local surgical and orthopaedic patients;

    (4)  Patients transferred from cardiac stepdown units;

    (5)  Patients receiving total parenteral nutrition;

    (6)  Patients with chronic renal failure who may need hemodialysis.

5. Limitations:

  a. 8 West has only 8 private rooms for the isolation of patients with infectious diseases or reduced resistance to disease.

  b. The unit is staffed and designed for the acutely ill adult patient as outlined above, not the critically ill adult, not the pediatric patient. Generally, patients under 15 years of age will not be admitted to 8 West. If such a patient is admitted, he will be considered a boarder. Other patients who are not candidates for admission to 8 West include:

    (1)  Acutely ill obstetric/gynecological patients;

    (2)  Patients requiring cardiac monitoring, intracardiac invasive monitoring, or peritoneal dialysis;

(3) Patients requiring endotracheal intubation ventilator management. Tracheostomy and oropharangeal airways may be managed on the unit, however;

(4) Patients requiring titrated medications to control vital functions, such as antihypertensives, inotropic agents, or antiarrhythmics;

(5) Patients having acute psychotic episodes, including drug and alcohol withdrawal.

c. Patients requiring diagnostic testing may be temporarily placed in the 8 West treatment room; patients from other units placed in the treatment room will be managed by the nursing staff from those units during the testing. Treatment room appointments can be made through the nursing management team.

6. Demand for Beds Beyond Capacity:

a. The capacity of 8 West is 40 beds. When the patient census exceeds the budgeted daily census, the shift coordinator will notify the PCS or NOS.

b. The shift coordinator will consult the admissions office early each day to validate potential or scheduled discharges and anticipated admissions. She will also collaborate with the admission office on determining the number, time of admission, and placement of patients.

c. If the admissions office or the emergency room need to place a patient on 8 West and no bed is available, the shift coordinator and admitting officer will collaborate with the Chief of Service to transfer or discharge an appropriate 8 West patient. The NOS will address staffing needs accordingly.

B. Length of Stay:

1. Generally, length of stay is determined by the patient's physical status and his ability to perform self care, as determined by the attending physician and the nursing staff.

2. A patient's length of stay should be consistent with the average stay for 8 West patients with similar conditions and acuity levels. The attending physician and the nursing staff will maintain quality care so that the patient can be discharged as early as possible.

3. All available resources should be used to facilitate a timely discharge—for example, social services, patient discharge preparation rounds, daily interaction between the doctor and family.

4. All patients with extended lengths of stay will be noted by the PCS and shift coordinator, and reported weekly to the Utilization Review Committee. Periodic care conferences shall determine priorities for these patients and plan their care accordingly.

5. The attending physician will justify an extended length of stay in the patient's medical record.

C. Discharge/Transfer Policies:

1. Patients can be discharged only by written or oral order of the attending physician.

2. The nursing staff, with the cooperation of the admitting officer, may transfer a patient at its discretion for the welfare of the patient, his family, or the nursing unit in general. Before this is done, every attempt must be made by the nursing staff to contact the attending physician. If the attending physician cannot be contacted, the admissions office will advise him of the transfer as soon as possible.

3. Patients will be assessed daily as to their continued hospitalization and their transfer or discharge status. The responsible RN and the attending physician will collaborate on the daily assessment. The patient's status will be recorded on the *Discharge/Transfer Planning Documentation Record* as well as in the medical progress notes.

4. Discharge planning rounds will be held weekly on 8 West. The PCS, shift coordinator, staff members, and representatives from the dietary, social services, and other departments as invited will attend. The purpose of discharge planning rounds is to review the status of each patient on the unit and discuss plans for assisting patients and families to meet physical, psychological, and cognitive requirements for discharge. The nursing staff will prepare for these rounds by assessing the needs of their patients and families as well as requirements for discharge.

5. If a patient is to be discharged to another institution, the responsible RN will talk to the patient's doctor about whether a nurse should accompany the patient. The department of nursing policy on "Institutional Transfer of Patients" explains how this should be done. (Refer to generic Department of Nursing Structure Standards.) Whether a nurse accompanies the patient or not, an updated care plan and a copy of the patient's record must always go with him.

6. Discharges will be documented in the 8 West log by the RN responsible for discharging the patient or as delegated to the unit clerk.

7. Discharge Criteria from 8 West are:

   a. The patient achieves independence from life support equipment, such as peritoneal dialysis, IV therapy, indwelling lines, unless sent home with supportive care.

   b. The patient achieves independence from therapeutic measures performed by nursing or support services, unless continued at home with assistance.

   c. The patient achieves stable body systems and physiologic parameters.

   d. The patient achieves stable laboratory values that have a bearing on his diagnostics.

   e. The patient and his family have shown they have coped reasonably well with his illness or injury.

   f. The patient and his family have demonstrated post discharge care and its implementation, with or without assistance.

## VII. GOVERNING RULES OF THE UNIT:

A. General Safety:

1. Visitor Traffic Control:

   a. Visiting hours and regulations on 8 West will be the same as those specified in department of nursing and hospital policies.

   b. The nursing staff on the unit may alter these visiting hours and regulations at its discretion, as warranted by the patient's condition. Security personnel are available to help control visitors.

   c. The unit is not to be used by hospital employees for social visits. Only patients, visitors, doctors, nurses, and other health care workers engaged in patient care should be on the unit. Neither is 8 West to be used as a thru traffic area.

2. Private duty Nurses and Students:

   a. When private duty nurses are assigned to patients on 8 West, the nursing staff will supervise the care they deliver. The unit's full-time nurses will also work with private duty nurses to see that their level of care is up to quality standards. For specific limitations on private duty nurses, see the department of nursing policy (Addendum H).

    b. The nursing management team for 8 West will adhere to the department of nursing policy on affiliation with nursing schools as well as the specific roles of nursing students working on the unit (see Addendum I).

    c. All patients assigned to nursing students will also be assigned to an RN who will be responsible for the overall welfare of the patient.

3. Smoking Restrictions:

    a. No smoking will be permitted at the nursing station. Smoking will be allowed in the employee lounges only. Patients assigned to rooms in which oxygen has been installed will be instructed that they are not allowed to smoke in their rooms.

    b. "No Smoking" signs will be posted in the rooms of all patients receiving oxygen.

4. In all other general safety matters, 8 West follows the department of nursing policy (see Addendum A).

B. Electrical Safety and Maintenance:

1. The Biomedical Department will perform regularly scheduled maintenance on portable defibrillators and monitors, electrical beds, diagnostic equipment, EKG machines, and other electrical equipment. Maintenance records will be kept by the PCS as part of 8 West Quality Assurance Activities and in the Biomedical Department.

2. When essential equipment malfunctions, it will be reported to the Biomedical Department immediately and the equipment itself labeled as out of order.

3. Nursing administration will arrange for malfunctioning equipment to be replaced when necessary.

4. Electrical safety standards for 8 West are summarized in Addendum B.

C. Infection Control:

1. 8 West adheres to the infection control measures outlined in the Department of Nursing Infection Control Manual. Patients requiring isolation precautions may be admitted to the unit only if a private room is available.

2. Specific infection control measures for 8 West may be found in Addendum C.

D. Patient Valuables:

1. Patient valuables are handled according to departmental and hospital policy.

2. Patients are discouraged from keeping jewelry or more than five dollars in cash in their rooms.

3. The patient's room will be kept neat and orderly by the nursing staff and his family.

4. Items necessary for the patient's convenience and comfort (such as eyeglasses, dentures, or prostheses) will be labeled with his name or placed in a container that is properly labeled.

E. Patient Confidentiality and Bill of Rights:

1. All patient information is confidential and is protected by the hospital's Patient Bill of Rights.

2. Any discussion of patient information in public areas is a violation of hospital policy, requiring disciplinary action.

3. Patient's records are to be seen only by the appropriate hospital employees.

4. Patients requesting to see their records may do so only in the presence of their doctor.

5. In accordance with hospital policy, nurses may not give out patient information to any news media unless prior arrangements have been made with the Nursing Administration and the Public Relation Department.

F. Emergency Equipment and Supplies:

1. Emergency equipment and supplies on 8 West include a crash cart, emergency drugs, and intubation equipment. Emergency trays can be found on the crash cart. See Addendum D for Crash Cart Checklist, see Addendum E for location on unit.

2. In an emergency, the EKG station or CCU will provide an EKG machine. A bedside monitor and defibrillator, located on the 8th floor, will be brought to the unit immediately during announced codes.

3. The crash cart is checked daily by the 8 West nursing staff and the check documented. The cart is located at the nursing station (see Addendum E for unit diagram showing location on nursing unit of carts, supplies, $O_2$ valves, emergency exits, fire extinguisher, fire alarms, and code Blue call buttons.) The crash cart is locked by disposable

system, with missing items replaced after each check. The disposable lock is then replaced.

4. After use, the crash cart will be exchanged for another in the CSR.

5. The NOS is responsible for providing backup supplies available for use in an emergency.

6. Other essential items of patient care are stocked on the unit. Stock medications are checked daily by the nursing staff and the pharmacy. The CSR cart is exchanged twice daily.

G. Patient Support Services:

1. 8 West has ready access to emergency and routine laboratory, diagnostic radiology, and blood bank services on a 24 hour basis. In accordance with department of nursing policy, the term *stat* will be reserved for life threatening or potential patient deterioration states as defined by the medical staff.

2. Any problems with support services on 8 West will be documented and discussed promptly for corrective action with the ADN, responsible service chief, and responsible department head. Additional policy on the interaction and roles of nursing personnel and support service staff may be found in generic department of nursing policy entitled "Clarification of Roles and Responsibilities for Nursing Staff and Support Personnel".

3. All patients have prompt access to hemodialysis as ordered by the physician. This may be accomplished by moving the patient to the dialysis unit or by intermittantly bringing the equipment to the patient's bedside. Details for logistics, safety, and role clarification between the 8 West nursing staff and dialysis staff may be found in generic department of nursing policy entitled "Hemodialysis In-house and Nursing Responsibilities".

H. Fire and Disaster Plans:

1. All staff will complete unit orientation related to the role of the nursing personnel and 8 West in hospital fire and disaster plans.

2. Additionally, all nursing personnel on 8 West will complete the annual fire and disaster drill conducted by the Hospital Safety Committee.

## VIII. STAFFING:

A. Quantity:

1. 8 West is staffed with enough professional and non-professional staff members to provide the required hours of nursing care for its average daily census, as outlined in the annual nursing budget.

2. The shift coordinator will classify patients by acuity levels before each shift and determine staffing needs accordingly.

3. The shift coordinator, PCS, and NOS will make arrangements to meet changing acuity levels or increased patient census. More nurses can be provided by approaching first part-time and then full-time staff to work overtime or by obtaining approved personnel available on a per diem basis through the NOS. Staff will also be floated to alternate unit when the other units staffing needs exceed those on 8 West. If alternate assignments are not needed, staff may be offered leave time. All staff will report to work as scheduled unless notified ahead of time by the unit POS or NOS. Required records of staff utilization will be maintained on the unit and in the nursing office. See Addendum E under Generic Structure for Department of Nursing for "Temporary Reassignment of Nursing Personnel and Records". The nursing office, working with PCS and the shift coordinator, will make any other staffing adjustments required on 8 West.

4. Staffing pattern (see Addendum F) is based on the above points as well as the department of nursing and personnel department policy on staffing.

5. The PCS is responsible for scheduling adequate nursing coverage of all patients on the unit. She must also adhere to the department of nursing policy that requires an RN to be assigned to each patient and to each non-professional staff member (such as LPN's and NA's) for appropriate direction and supervision. A staff scheduling committee makes the actual schedule, consistent with the staffing and scheduling policies for 8 West (see Addendum F). In the absence of the PCS, the shift coordinator will collaborate with the NOS to schedule current and upcoming shift coverage.

B. Levels:

1. Patient care on 8 West is given by the following:

   a. RN's;

   b. LPN's;

    c. NA's;

    d. private-duty nurses, either RN or LPN;

    e. clinical specialists;

    f. clinical instructors;

    g. student nurses.

2. All patients will have an RN assigned to them; all private-duty and student nurses, as well as the "float staff," will also have an RN assigned to them.

3. Staffing will always provide for no less than 75% regular unit staff at all times. Non-regular staff members will be assigned only to patients they're qualified to care for. They will not be made shift coordinator and will at all times work under the direction of the regular staff. They will receive an orientation to the unit and full report by the shift coordinator prior to giving patient cae.

4. Nursing students will be supervised by their instructor and the nursing staff on 8 West (see Addendum G).

C. Delivery of Care Method:

1. The method of delivering patient care on 8 West is consistent with the goals and philosophy of the department of nursing.

2. See Addendum H for policies addressing the following issues:

    a. Delivery of care method,

    b. RN responsibilities,

    c. Assignments,

    d. Reports,

    e. Charge nurse,

    f. Reponsibilities of non-professional staff.

3. See Addendum E for a unit diagram of the nursing teams.

D. Preparation:

1. Selection:

    a. Staff will be hired for 8 West by the PCS in collaboration with the ADN for Medical/Surgical Area. Staff will be selected based on current vacancies, education, experience, and an interview process (see Addendum I).

2. Orientation:

    a. All 8 West staff will complete hospital and unit orientation programs which are structured, formalized, and individualized.

    b. All staff will have an additional period of review at the end of the 3 week orientation period based on 8 West standards, nursing responsibilities for the specific patient population, and identified learning needs of the new staff member. All new graduates hired onto 8 West will complete the formal internship program in three months.

    c. See Addendum I for details.

3. Continuing Education:

    a. All staff will attend ongoing educational events held within the Department of Nursing and on 8 West. These educational activities will be based on routine and new responsibilities of nursing staff, identified learning needs, and data from patient care review activities.

    b. Mandatory educational activities are summarized in "Performance Standards for Growth and Development". Additionally, staff will attend all mandatory events dealing with the following issues:

        (1) CPR and Emergency Measures;

        (2) Safety, including General, Electrical, Fire, and Disaster;

        (3) Infection Control Review.

    c. Educational records will be maintained on 8 West; additionally, each staff member will maintain his own. The records will be reviewed annually at evaluation time. Participation in learning activities is an important part of the employee appraisal process as well as 8 West Quality Assurance Plans.

    d. See Addendum I.

4. Credentialing:

    a. All staff will be provided periodic assessments of learning needs, including surveys, questionnaires, and unsolicited suggestions for continuing education events.

    b. Staff will also complete Annual Internal Certification which will be conducted as a joint activity by Clinical Education, Clinical Specialists, and 8 West management team. Annual testing will be conducted to validate cognitive and skill knowledge required by the patient population on 8 West.

   c. Staff will complete ongoing Quality Assurance activities for the purpose of assuring compliance to unit standards, identifying learning needs, and identifying/resolving staff/unit/patient care problems.

## IX. NURSING RESPONSIBILITIES:

A. The professional staff (RN) on 8 West has these responsibilities:

1. General:

   a. All those responsibilities listed in generic department of nursing policies including the use of the nursing process when giving patient care.

   b. Use of physical and psychosocial assessment skills as specified in the units performance standards.

   c. Safe performance of all general medical/surgical procedures approved by the department of nursing.

   d. Timely and accurate reporting of abnormal diagnostic radiology and laboratory tests including pulmonary functions, blood and urine tests, xrays, and EKG.

   e. Timely and accurate reporting of significant changes in a patient's condition.

   f. Timely and accurate recording of physician's verbal orders.

   g. Implementation and evaluation of patient teaching and discharge activities as identified in unit protocols.

2. Psychomotor Skills:

   a. Administering IV push and continuous drip medications, as specified in department of nursing policy.

   b. Starting peripheral IV lines with physician's orders.

   c. Assisting with insertion of subclavian lines, cutdown catheters, and chest tubes.

   d. Removing subclavian and cutdown catheters.

   e. Changing chest tube drainage containers.

   f. Performing routine irrigations of nasogastric and gastrostomy tubes and Foley catheters, but not peripheral or central IV lines or chest tubes.

   g. Managing external shunts and Hickman catheters and assisting with declotting procedure.

h. Measuring CVP and managing the central line.

i. Aspirating blood for laboratory testing through a CVP line.

j. Cutting sutures for removal of a central line, but not putting them in or routinely removing wound sutures.

k. Maintaining a TPN line and performing care of the site.

3. Emergency Measures:

   a. Performing CPR as specified by the Resuscitation Committee.

   b. Implementing emergency protocol as specified in the unit's standards manual.

   c. Inserting an IV line with a needle or catheter and initiating 500cc D5W in potentially life-threatening situations.

   d. Replacing an established trachestomy tube (in place at least 72 hours) when it becomes dislodged.

   e. Inserting orpharyngeal airways, mushroom and trumpet airways.

B. The licensed practical nursing staff (LPN) has these responsibilities:

1. General:

   a. All those responsibilities listed in generic department of nursing policies.

   b. Use of physical and emotional observational skills as specified in the units performance standards.

   c. Safe performance of all general medical/surgical procedures approved for implementation by LPN's.

   d. Timely and accurate recording of physician's verbal orders.

   e. Direct patient care activities delegated by professional staff.

2. Psychomotor Skills:

   a. Routine hygiene measures of AM care, PM care, mouth/nose/eye care, back and skin routines, ROM.

   b. Irrigating nasogastric tubes.

   c. Inserting and irrigating Foley catheters.

   d. Attaching external (male) catheters.

e. Changing dressings on surgical wounds, peripheral and CVP IV's.

f. Starting peripheral IV's with needles or catheters.

g. Changing IV tubing for peripheral and central lines, but not TPN.

h. Hanging IV solutions without medications; hanging solutions mixed by pharmacy as directed.

i. Administering PO and IM medications.

j. Assisting in CPR basic and as directed by physicians and RN's.

k. Administering enemas and douches, and inserting rectal tubes.

l. Discontinuing peripheral IV lines.

m. Discontinuing nasogastric tubes and Foley catheters.

n. Stripping chest tubes.

APPROVED: November 1982
8 West Head Nurse/Nursing Staff
Director of Nursing
Review: November 1987
Revision: November 1986
Distribution: 8W Standards Manual

# HOSPITAL
## DEPARTMENT OF NURSING
### ORGANIZATIONAL CHART FOR UNIT 8 WEST

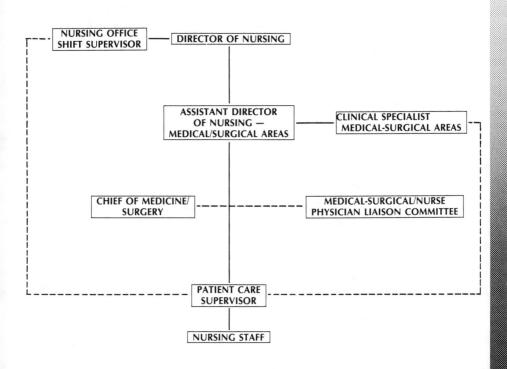

———————— Direct line responsibility
— — — — — — Collaborative/communicative responsibility

APPROVED: November 1982
8 West PCS
Nursing Staff
Review: November 1987
Revision: November 1986

# NARRATIVE

The foundation of the organizational structure of the Medical/Surgical unit, 8 West is the Patient Care Supervisor (PCS). She is responsible for the daily operation of the nursing unit and for daily coordination and collaboration with the medical staff as well as with other Department Heads and the Nursing Service Administration. Her position carries the authority to identify and work toward resolution of problems affecting her unit both directly and indirectly in all clinical and managerial areas. Her authority is both informal within her peer group for analysis and decision making and formal through interaction with the Assistant Director of Nursing (ADN) and other members of the Nursing Management Team.

Further, the PCS is responsible for implementing all the elements outlined in the PCS job description and performance standards. Her focus is the direction and development of the nursing staff through standards and participative supervisory methods and the maintenance of an efficiently running nursing unit. Her overall goal of optimum patient care is achieved through the development of annual unit goals which spring from those of the Department of Nursing. She works closely with the Assistant Director for Medical Surgical Areas in the creative resolution of issues, development of standards, and Quality Assurance activities.

The nursing staff on 8 West consists of both professional and nonprofessional staff members. Professional staff will be on the unit at all times in sufficient numbers to assume responsibility for directing, planning, and evaluating patient care using the nursing process. All patients on the unit are assigned to RN's and RN staff is assigned responsibility for the non professional staff members, consisting of licensed practical nurses and nursing assistants. A "charge" RN is designated for each shift. RN's have total patient care assignments and are responsible for both the continuity and quality of care delivered to their patients. All staff are expected to participate in the affairs of the unit such as unit goal achievement, standards development and implementation, and quality assurance activities.

The PCS reports directly to the ADN of Medical Surgical Areas who in turn reports directly to the Director of Nursing. The ADN is responsible for the supervision and development of the PCS and serves as a resource person and role model while assisting the PCS in the dissemination of communication, establishment and implementation of unit/department objectives, unit policy and standards, and staff development.

The Clinical Specialist (Medical Surgical Areas) is an advanced practitioner in a non-line position responsible for the clinical role modeling for the nursing staff. She participates in problem identification on the unit in relation to clinical issues and assists with clinical development of the staff and standards development. The clinical instructor is in a collaborative role to facilitate the effective orientation of new staff members to the unit and to function interdependently with the clinical specialist in the meeting of staff learning needs.

The Nursing Officer Supervisor (NOS) functions in a line position on the alternate shifts (evenings and night) as a supervisor for staff and patient care as well as an administrative support and resource person to assigned units. Her responsibilities focus on ongoing implementation of nursing service, hospital, and unit standards, identification and communication of problems, and participation in resolution methods.

Both the PCS and ADN are in a collaborative role with the President of the Medical Staff and Chiefs of the various services of patients admitted to 8 West. Both members of the nursing administrative team are expected to maintain open lines of communication and high level working relationships with these designated physician leaders for the purpose of problem identification and problem resolution. The PCS and ADN attend the quarterly Physician Liaison Committee meeting to facilitate effective working relationships between the medical and nursing staffs.

# ADDENDUM A

## Nursing Safety Policy

A. Patient Identification:

1. Patients will wear an identification band on the wrist or ankle at all times. If a patient's physical condition prevents this, then the band will be taped on the arm or leg.

2. Patients will be identified properly before receiving medications, as specified in the hospital and department of nursing policy on medication administration. Patient identification will be conducted in the same manner before blood administration.

B. Beds:

1. Beds will be in the low position at all times unless the side rails are up or a nurse is with the patient, giving hands-on care.

2. Call lights will be placed within reach of all patients, whether they're in bed or sitting in a chair.

3. All patients will be shown how to use bedside and bathroom call lights, and instructed not to lock bathroom doors.

4. Side rails will be raised under the following circumstances (unless the patient or his family has released the hospital from this responsibility):

   • at bedtime;

   • following the administration of sedatives or narcotics;

   • when the patient is confused or found to have some other alteration in level of consciousness.

C. Transport:

1. The wheels on all beds, wheelchairs, and stretchers will be locked when not being used to transport a patient or when the patient is not being attended to by a nurse.

2. At least two people are needed to push a stretcher or bed occupied by a patient.

3. All IV's must be suspended from IV poles during transport.

4. Patients being transported on stretchers must be secured with both straps.

5. All wheelchairs will be backed into elevators.

D. Restraints:

1. Restraints may not be applied without a doctor's order. In an emergency, Posey or soft wrist restraints may be applied while ' ·~r is being called. In such cases, a nurse or family

member must remain with the patient until the doctor's order has been obtained and charted.

2. At no time will restraints be tied to side rails.

3. If a patient requires full side rails on his bed, the Biomedical Department will be contacted; double short side rails may not be substituted.

E. Smoking:

1. In accordance with hospital policy, patients are only allowed to smoke in the solariums.

Approved: 9/84
           Safety Committee
           Department of Nursing

Review: 9/87

Revision: 9/86

# ADDENDUM B

## Electrical Safety Policy

1. "Cheater" or multiple adaptors will not be used on nursing units. Extension cords (no longer than 10 feet) may be used only in an emergency.

2. Disconnect plugs from wall sockets by grasping the plug itself, not the cord.

3. All electrical equipment used in patient care requires a three-pronged hospital safety plug and a three-wire power cord receptacle.

4. When a patient is connected to more than one piece of electrical equipment, adjacent receptacles must be used to reduce the risk of creating different ground potentials or electrical shock hazards.

5. Don't use any piece of electrical equipment if:

   - it's been dropped or otherwise damaged.
   - it's given someone an electrical shock.
   - it smells or feels like it's overheating.
   - liquid has been spilled on it.

   Report any piece of damaged electrical equipment immediately to the appropriate department. Label it and promptly remove it from the patient area.

6. Report any wire or cord that's frayed, worn, burned, cut, or warm during use to the Biomedical Department. Also report any plug that's broken, bent, or has loose prongs; any receptacles that don't fit into the wall properly, don't grip the plug securely, or don't supply enough power; and any equipment with knobs or switches that are loose or don't turn properly.

7. When using an EKG machine to introduce a pacemaker catheter, always connect the catheter to the V-lead of the EKG machine. Don't let anyone or anything that's grounded come in contact with the V-lead electrode terminal. Always use a gloved hand to touch exposed electrode wires. Keep the terminals or pacemaker catheter covered with nonconductive material (such as a rubber glove or plastic bag) at all times during use. Report poor quality tracing (such as slanted, out of focus, dim, or off-center tracing, or excessive blinking) and any 60-cycle interference to the Biomedical Department.

8. In accordance with hospital policy, no electrical appliances not approved by the Biomedical Department may be brought into a patient's room. Examples would be hair dryers or hot plates.

# ADDENDUM C

## Infection Control Policy for 8 West

While it is understood that the nursing staff will follow the general hospital policy on infection control, more specific measures will also be carried out on 8 West. Strict adherance to infection control policy is particularly important on this unit because so many of its patients are elderly and debilitated. Some are receiving chemotherapeutic drugs or have fevers of unknown origin or overt infections that also make prevention of cross-contamination essential.

Specific infection control policies to be carried out on 8 West are:

1. Personnel:

   A. Personnel working on the unit will not report for work with a fever, diarrhea, or an infection of the skin or upper respiratory tract.

   B. Employees with these conditions must see the hospital's employee nurse or doctor.

2. Attire:

   A. Each unit member will wear clean professional attire for direct patient care.

   B. Unit members may not wear sweaters during direct patient care. Unit members will follow the dress code.

3. Handwashing:

   A. Handwashing, one of the most effective infection control measures, is required between contact with patients and between procedures.

4. Invasive Equipment:

   A. Suction devices:

   - Change suction tubing and reusable or disposible cannisters every 8 hours.

   - Send all reusable equipment for cleaning and sterilization every 24 hours.

   - Perform all tracheostomy or respiratory care and suctioning strictly according to procedure and protocol.

   - Place all contaminated items, such as catheters and tissues, in a plastic bag. Seal the bag securely and dispose of it in a plastic lined waste basket.

   B. Catheter insertion, irrigation, and maintenance (see procedures, such as "Foley catheter insertion").

C. Registered nurses should obtain cultures of any wound drainage that appears abnormal in color, odor, or other characteristics. Obtain a physician order afterwards.

D. RN staff will collaborate with the medical staff on obtaining follow-up cultures so that the effectiveness of treatment can be evaluated.

E. All staff will use the smallest solution container possible when irrigating invasive equipment. Discard the container after one use; use each irrigation set once only.

F. Dressing changes:

- Wear gloves during all dressing changes.

- Wear a mask for TPN dressing changes.

- Change pacemaker and peripheral line dressings every other day; change TPN and central line dressings every day. Change routing surgical dressings PRN (at least daily) unless ordered otherwise.

G. Draining wounds:

- Culture draining wounds as described above.

- Isolate pathological drainage as specified in the Infection Control Manual.

- "Bag" draining wounds to control excessive drainage; perform skin care measures as ordered by the doctor, enterostomal therapist, or infection control nurse.

5. Isolation Precautions:

A. Perform isolation precautions as specified in the Infection Control Manual.

B. Place the infectious patient in a private room; post precautionary signs on the door and over the bed.

C. Obtain infection control supplies and equipment from the CSR. Place in the room, use for that patient only, and clean terminally afterwards.

D. Notify the dietary and radiology departments, as well as the pharmacy and lab, of the patient's condition. Advise them to take appropriate actions.

E. Notify the infection control nurse of all known or suspected cases of infection on 8 West.

6. Housekeeping:

A. Mop the unit twice a week with disinfectant as specified in the Infection Control Manual.

B. Replace semiprivate curtains every month.

C. Disinfect patient's bed and bedside equipment after discharge.

D. Housekeeping personnel will disinfect all rooms occupied by infectious patients.

APPROVED: 6/82
        PCS/8 West Nursing Staff
        Infection Control Committee
        Department of Nursing

REVIEW: 6/87

REVISION: 6/86

# ADDENDUM D

## DEPARTMENT OF NURSING

UNIT:

DATE INITIATED:

DATE COMPLETED:

## EMERGENCY CART CHECK LIST

*Instructions:*
Maintain in unit QA Manual and summarize on Unit QA Report; return all used forms to Staff Development.

| | DATE: | 1 | 2 | 3 | 4 | 5 | 6 | 7 | 8 | 9 | 10 | 11 | 12 | 13 | 14 | 15 | 16 | 17 | 18 | 19 | 20 | 21 | 22 | 23 | 24 | 25 | 26 | 27 | 28 | 29 | 30 | 31 |
|---|---|---|---|---|---|---|---|---|---|---|---|---|---|---|---|---|---|---|---|---|---|---|---|---|---|---|---|---|---|---|---|---|
| | RESPIRATORY EQUIP. | | | | | | | | | | | | | | | | | | | | | | | | | | | | | | | |
| | TOP BOXTRAY: | | | | | | | | | | | | | | | | | | | | | | | | | | | | | | | |
| | Laryngoscope | | | | | | | | | | | | | | | | | | | | | | | | | | | | | | | |
| | #3 curved blade | | | | | | | | | | | | | | | | | | | | | | | | | | | | | | | |
| | #4 curved blade | | | | | | | | | | | | | | | | | | | | | | | | | | | | | | | |
| | 5 in one connector | | | | | | | | | | | | | | | | | | | | | | | | | | | | | | | |
| | Straight blade | | | | | | | | | | | | | | | | | | | | | | | | | | | | | | | |
| | McGill Forceps | | | | | | | | | | | | | | | | | | | | | | | | | | | | | | | |
| 1 | 10cc syringe | | | | | | | | | | | | | | | | | | | | | | | | | | | | | | | |
| 2 | Batteries | | | | | | | | | | | | | | | | | | | | | | | | | | | | | | | |
| 2 | Bulbs | | | | | | | | | | | | | | | | | | | | | | | | | | | | | | | |
| 1 | Guide wire | | | | | | | | | | | | | | | | | | | | | | | | | | | | | | | |
| 1 | Xylocaine Ointment | | | | | | | | | | | | | | | | | | | | | | | | | | | | | | | |
| 1 | Large K.Y. Jelly | | | | | | | | | | | | | | | | | | | | | | | | | | | | | | | |
| 1 | Adult airway (small) | | | | | | | | | | | | | | | | | | | | | | | | | | | | | | | |
| 1 | Adult airway (large) | | | | | | | | | | | | | | | | | | | | | | | | | | | | | | | |
| 1 | Adult airway (medium) | | | | | | | | | | | | | | | | | | | | | | | | | | | | | | | |
| 1 | Padded Tongue Blades | | | | | | | | | | | | | | | | | | | | | | | | | | | | | | | |
| 1 | Roll 2" Cloth Tape | | | | | | | | | | | | | | | | | | | | | | | | | | | | | | | |
| 2 | Packages Benzoin | | | | | | | | | | | | | | | | | | | | | | | | | | | | | | | |
| | Disposable scissors | | | | | | | | | | | | | | | | | | | | | | | | | | | | | | | |
| 1 | 5 in 1 connector | | | | | | | | | | | | | | | | | | | | | | | | | | | | | | | |
| | BOTTOM: | | | | | | | | | | | | | | | | | | | | | | | | | | | | | | | |
| 1 | #5 Tracheal tube | | | | | | | | | | | | | | | | | | | | | | | | | | | | | | | |
| 1 | #6 Tracheal tube | | | | | | | | | | | | | | | | | | | | | | | | | | | | | | | |
| 2 | #7 Tracheal tube | | | | | | | | | | | | | | | | | | | | | | | | | | | | | | | |
| 2 | #8 Tracheal tube | | | | | | | | | | | | | | | | | | | | | | | | | | | | | | | |
| 2 | #9 Tracheal tube | | | | | | | | | | | | | | | | | | | | | | | | | | | | | | | |
| | Initials: | | | | | | | | | | | | | | | | | | | | | | | | | | | | | | | |

| | DATE: | 1 | 2 | 3 | 4 | 5 | 6 | 7 | 8 | 9 | 10 | 11 | 12 | 13 | 14 | 15 | 16 | 17 | 18 | 19 | 20 | 21 | 22 | 23 | 24 | 25 | 26 | 27 | 28 | 29 | 30 | 31 |
|---|---|---|---|---|---|---|---|---|---|---|---|---|---|---|---|---|---|---|---|---|---|---|---|---|---|---|---|---|---|---|---|---|
| 2 | Suction catheters #14 (kit) | | | | | | | | | | | | | | | | | | | | | | | | | | | | | | | |
| 2 | Suction catheters #12 | | | | | | | | | | | | | | | | | | | | | | | | | | | | | | | |
| 1 | Tonsil suction | | | | | | | | | | | | | | | | | | | | | | | | | | | | | | | |
| 1 | Adult $O_2$ mask | | | | | | | | | | | | | | | | | | | | | | | | | | | | | | | |
| 1 | Suction extension set | | | | | | | | | | | | | | | | | | | | | | | | | | | | | | | |
| 1 | $O_2$ Nasal prongs | | | | | | | | | | | | | | | | | | | | | | | | | | | | | | | |
| | DRAWER #1 (Right side) | | | | | | | | | | | | | | | | | | | | | | | | | | | | | | | |
| 6 | Sodium Bicarb Bristojets | | | | | | | | | | | | | | | | | | | | | | | | | | | | | | | |
| 2 | Calcium Bristojets | | | | | | | | | | | | | | | | | | | | | | | | | | | | | | | |
| 2 | Lidocaine Bristojets | | | | | | | | | | | | | | | | | | | | | | | | | | | | | | | |
| 2 | Atropine Bristojets | | | | | | | | | | | | | | | | | | | | | | | | | | | | | | | |
| 2 | Epinephrine 1:10,000 in 10cc | | | | | | | | | | | | | | | | | | | | | | | | | | | | | | | |
| 1 | Bristojets Intra cardiac) | | | | | | | | | | | | | | | | | | | | | | | | | | | | | | | |
| 2 | Valium 10mg Bristojets | | | | | | | | | | | | | | | | | | | | | | | | | | | | | | | |
| 1 | 50% Dextrose Bristojet | | | | | | | | | | | | | | | | | | | | | | | | | | | | | | | |
| | DRAWER #1 (Left side) | | | | | | | | | | | | | | | | | | | | | | | | | | | | | | | |
| 2 | Aminophyllin (500mg) amp | | | | | | | | | | | | | | | | | | | | | | | | | | | | | | | |
| 1 | Benadryl 50mg tubex | | | | | | | | | | | | | | | | | | | | | | | | | | | | | | | |
| 2 | Bretylol (Bretyllium 500mg) | | | | | | | | | | | | | | | | | | | | | | | | | | | | | | | |
| 1 | Digoxin | | | | | | | | | | | | | | | | | | | | | | | | | | | | | | | |
| 4 | Dilantin 250mg amps | | | | | | | | | | | | | | | | | | | | | | | | | | | | | | | |
| 2 | Epinephrine amps 1:000 | | | | | | | | | | | | | | | | | | | | | | | | | | | | | | | |
| 5 | Inderal (1mg) amps | | | | | | | | | | | | | | | | | | | | | | | | | | | | | | | |
| 2 | Isuprel (1mg) amps | | | | | | | | | | | | | | | | | | | | | | | | | | | | | | | |
| 2 | Ephedrine 50mg amps | | | | | | | | | | | | | | | | | | | | | | | | | | | | | | | |
| 3 | Lasix (40mg) amps | | | | | | | | | | | | | | | | | | | | | | | | | | | | | | | |
| 2 | Levophed amps (4mgs) | | | | | | | | | | | | | | | | | | | | | | | | | | | | | | | |
| 4 | Narcan, prefilled syringes | | | | | | | | | | | | | | | | | | | | | | | | | | | | | | | |
| 2 | Verapamil, amps | | | | | | | | | | | | | | | | | | | | | | | | | | | | | | | |
| 3 | Pronestyl (100mg) amps | | | | | | | | | | | | | | | | | | | | | | | | | | | | | | | |
| | Initials: | | | | | | | | | | | | | | | | | | | | | | | | | | | | | | | |

| | DATE: | 1 | 2 | 3 | 4 | 5 | 6 | 7 | 8 | 9 | 10 | 11 | 12 | 13 | 14 | 15 | 16 | 17 | 18 | 19 | 20 | 21 | 22 | 23 | 24 | 25 | 26 | 27 | 28 | 29 | 30 | 31 |
|---|---|---|---|---|---|---|---|---|---|---|---|---|---|---|---|---|---|---|---|---|---|---|---|---|---|---|---|---|---|---|---|---|
| | DRAWER #2 | | | | | | | | | | | | | | | | | | | | | | | | | | | | | | | |
| 1 | 500 cc D5W with Lidocaine | | | | | | | | | | | | | | | | | | | | | | | | | | | | | | | |
| | (2 Gm) Bristojets attached | | | | | | | | | | | | | | | | | | | | | | | | | | | | | | | |
| 1 | 500cc D5W with Dopamine | | | | | | | | | | | | | | | | | | | | | | | | | | | | | | | |
| | (800mg) Bristojets attached | | | | | | | | | | | | | | | | | | | | | | | | | | | | | | | |
| 2 | Mini drop solu. adm. sets (McGaw) | | | | | | | | | | | | | | | | | | | | | | | | | | | | | | | |
| | | | | | | | | | | | | | | | | | | | | | | | | | | | | | | | | |
| 2 | Sterile H$_2$O (10cc) fr irrig | | | | | | | | | | | | | | | | | | | | | | | | | | | | | | | |
| 2 | Sterile N/S (10cc) fr irrig | | | | | | | | | | | | | | | | | | | | | | | | | | | | | | | |
| 1 | Box alcohol swabs | | | | | | | | | | | | | | | | | | | | | | | | | | | | | | | |
| 5 | Red labels for IV additive | | | | | | | | | | | | | | | | | | | | | | | | | | | | | | | |
| 1 | Roll 1" Plastic Tape | | | | | | | | | | | | | | | | | | | | | | | | | | | | | | | |
| | Syringes: | | | | | | | | | | | | | | | | | | | | | | | | | | | | | | | |
| 5 | 3cc with needles | | | | | | | | | | | | | | | | | | | | | | | | | | | | | | | |
| 5 | 5cc with 20 g. needle | | | | | | | | | | | | | | | | | | | | | | | | | | | | | | | |
| 5 | 10cc | | | | | | | | | | | | | | | | | | | | | | | | | | | | | | | |
| 2 | 20cc | | | | | | | | | | | | | | | | | | | | | | | | | | | | | | | |
| 2 | 30cc | | | | | | | | | | | | | | | | | | | | | | | | | | | | | | | |
| 1 | 60cc | | | | | | | | | | | | | | | | | | | | | | | | | | | | | | | |
| | Needles: | | | | | | | | | | | | | | | | | | | | | | | | | | | | | | | |
| 5 | 22 g 1" | | | | | | | | | | | | | | | | | | | | | | | | | | | | | | | |
| 5 | 20 g 1" | | | | | | | | | | | | | | | | | | | | | | | | | | | | | | | |
| 5 | 18 g 1" | | | | | | | | | | | | | | | | | | | | | | | | | | | | | | | |
| | | | | | | | | | | | | | | | | | | | | | | | | | | | | | | | | |
| | Spinal Needles: | | | | | | | | | | | | | | | | | | | | | | | | | | | | | | | |
| 2 | 20 g 3½" | | | | | | | | | | | | | | | | | | | | | | | | | | | | | | | |
| 2 | 22 g 3½" | | | | | | | | | | | | | | | | | | | | | | | | | | | | | | | |
| 2 | 18 g 3½" | | | | | | | | | | | | | | | | | | | | | | | | | | | | | | | |
| | | | | | | | | | | | | | | | | | | | | | | | | | | | | | | | | |
| | | | | | | | | | | | | | | | | | | | | | | | | | | | | | | | | |
| | | | | | | | | | | | | | | | | | | | | | | | | | | | | | | | | |
| | Initials: | | | | | | | | | | | | | | | | | | | | | | | | | | | | | | | |

| | DATE: | 1 | 2 | 3 | 4 | 5 | 6 | 7 | 8 | 9 | 10 | 11 | 12 | 13 | 14 | 15 | 16 | 17 | 18 | 19 | 20 | 21 | 22 | 23 | 24 | 25 | 26 | 27 | 28 | 29 | 30 | 31 |
|---|---|---|---|---|---|---|---|---|---|---|---|---|---|---|---|---|---|---|---|---|---|---|---|---|---|---|---|---|---|---|---|---|
| | DRAWER #3 | | | | | | | | | | | | | | | | | | | | | | | | | | | | | | | |
| 1 | Prep Tray | | | | | | | | | | | | | | | | | | | | | | | | | | | | | | | |
| 1 | BP cuff & stethoscope | | | | | | | | | | | | | | | | | | | | | | | | | | | | | | | |
| 1 | N/G (sump) tube #16 Fr. | | | | | | | | | | | | | | | | | | | | | | | | | | | | | | | |
| 2 | Connecting tubings | | | | | | | | | | | | | | | | | | | | | | | | | | | | | | | |
| 1 | Piston (Toomey) syringe | | | | | | | | | | | | | | | | | | | | | | | | | | | | | | | |
| 1 | Roll 1″ adhesive tape | | | | | | | | | | | | | | | | | | | | | | | | | | | | | | | |
| 5 | Benzoin Swabs | | | | | | | | | | | | | | | | | | | | | | | | | | | | | | | |
| 2 | Arterial blood gas kits | | | | | | | | | | | | | | | | | | | | | | | | | | | | | | | |
| | DRAWER #4 | | | | | | | | | | | | | | | | | | | | | | | | | | | | | | | |
| 1 | Cut down tray | | | | | | | | | | | | | | | | | | | | | | | | | | | | | | | |
| 1 | Sterile Instrument Pack | | | | | | | | | | | | | | | | | | | | | | | | | | | | | | | |
| 1 | Cordis (1g. bore cath.) | | | | | | | | | | | | | | | | | | | | | | | | | | | | | | | |
| | Gloves: | | | | | | | | | | | | | | | | | | | | | | | | | | | | | | | |
| 2 | Size 6 | | | | | | | | | | | | | | | | | | | | | | | | | | | | | | | |
| 2 | Size 7 | | | | | | | | | | | | | | | | | | | | | | | | | | | | | | | |
| 2 | Size 7½ | | | | | | | | | | | | | | | | | | | | | | | | | | | | | | | |
| 2 | Size 8 | | | | | | | | | | | | | | | | | | | | | | | | | | | | | | | |
| | Betadine solu (10cc) | | | | | | | | | | | | | | | | | | | | | | | | | | | | | | | |
| 3 | Benzoin Swabs | | | | | | | | | | | | | | | | | | | | | | | | | | | | | | | |
| 1 | Roll 2″ adhesive tape | | | | | | | | | | | | | | | | | | | | | | | | | | | | | | | |
| | DRAWER #5 | | | | | | | | | | | | | | | | | | | | | | | | | | | | | | | |
| 1 | 1000cc 5D/W | | | | | | | | | | | | | | | | | | | | | | | | | | | | | | | |
| 2 | 500cc 5D/W | | | | | | | | | | | | | | | | | | | | | | | | | | | | | | | |
| 1 | 1000cc N/S | | | | | | | | | | | | | | | | | | | | | | | | | | | | | | | |
| | | | | | | | | | | | | | | | | | | | | | | | | | | | | | | | | |
| 1 | 1000cc Lac. Ringers | | | | | | | | | | | | | | | | | | | | | | | | | | | | | | | |
| 2 | Mini-drip solu adm. sets | | | | | | | | | | | | | | | | | | | | | | | | | | | | | | | |
| 4 | Macro-drip solu adm. sets | | | | | | | | | | | | | | | | | | | | | | | | | | | | | | | |
| 4 | I.V. extension sets | | | | | | | | | | | | | | | | | | | | | | | | | | | | | | | |
| | | | | | | | | | | | | | | | | | | | | | | | | | | | | | | | | |
| | Initials: | | | | | | | | | | | | | | | | | | | | | | | | | | | | | | | |

| | DATE: | 1 | 2 | 3 | 4 | 5 | 6 | 7 | 8 | 9 | 10 | 11 | 12 | 13 | 14 | 15 | 16 | 17 | 18 | 19 | 20 | 21 | 22 | 23 | 24 | 25 | 26 | 27 | 28 | 29 | 30 | 31 |
|---|---|---|---|---|---|---|---|---|---|---|---|---|---|---|---|---|---|---|---|---|---|---|---|---|---|---|---|---|---|---|---|---|
| | DRAWER #5 (continued) | | | | | | | | | | | | | | | | | | | | | | | | | | | | | | | |
| 5 | 2 × 2's | | | | | | | | | | | | | | | | | | | | | | | | | | | | | | | |
| 5 | 4 × 4's | | | | | | | | | | | | | | | | | | | | | | | | | | | | | | | |
| 5 | Betadine Swabs | | | | | | | | | | | | | | | | | | | | | | | | | | | | | | | |
| 1 | Roll 1″ adhesive tape | | | | | | | | | | | | | | | | | | | | | | | | | | | | | | | |
| 2 | Tourniquets | | | | | | | | | | | | | | | | | | | | | | | | | | | | | | | |
| 1 | Long arm board | | | | | | | | | | | | | | | | | | | | | | | | | | | | | | | |
| 1 | Short arm board | | | | | | | | | | | | | | | | | | | | | | | | | | | | | | | |
| 5 | Red medication labels | | | | | | | | | | | | | | | | | | | | | | | | | | | | | | | |
| | Butterfly I.V. Needles: | | | | | | | | | | | | | | | | | | | | | | | | | | | | | | | |
| 2 | 23 gauge | | | | | | | | | | | | | | | | | | | | | | | | | | | | | | | |
| 2 | 21 gauge | | | | | | | | | | | | | | | | | | | | | | | | | | | | | | | |
| 2 | 19 gauge | | | | | | | | | | | | | | | | | | | | | | | | | | | | | | | |
| | | | | | | | | | | | | | | | | | | | | | | | | | | | | | | | | |
| | Angio caths: | | | | | | | | | | | | | | | | | | | | | | | | | | | | | | | |
| 2 | 22 gauge - 1″ | | | | | | | | | | | | | | | | | | | | | | | | | | | | | | | |
| 2 | 20 gauge - 1″ | | | | | | | | | | | | | | | | | | | | | | | | | | | | | | | |
| 2 | 18 gauge - 2″ | | | | | | | | | | | | | | | | | | | | | | | | | | | | | | | |
| 2 | 16 gauge - 2″ | | | | | | | | | | | | | | | | | | | | | | | | | | | | | | | |
| 2 | 14 gauge - 2″ | | | | | | | | | | | | | | | | | | | | | | | | | | | | | | | |
| | | | | | | | | | | | | | | | | | | | | | | | | | | | | | | | | |
| | MISCELLANEOUS: | | | | | | | | | | | | | | | | | | | | | | | | | | | | | | | |
| 2 | CVP catheters (taped to side of cart) | | | | | | | | | | | | | | | | | | | | | | | | | | | | | | | |
| 1 | Electric suction machine | | | | | | | | | | | | | | | | | | | | | | | | | | | | | | | |
| | (bottom shelf of cart) | | | | | | | | | | | | | | | | | | | | | | | | | | | | | | | |
| 1 | Ambu bag with mask | | | | | | | | | | | | | | | | | | | | | | | | | | | | | | | |
| 1 | $O_2$ Flow meter | | | | | | | | | | | | | | | | | | | | | | | | | | | | | | | |
| 1 | $O_2$ connecting tube | | | | | | | | | | | | | | | | | | | | | | | | | | | | | | | |
| | Needle Box | | | | | | | | | | | | | | | | | | | | | | | | | | | | | | | |
| 1 | Suction bottle | | | | | | | | | | | | | | | | | | | | | | | | | | | | | | | |
| 1 | Suction connecting tube | | | | | | | | | | | | | | | | | | | | | | | | | | | | | | | |
| | Initials: | | | | | | | | | | | | | | | | | | | | | | | | | | | | | | | |

| DATE: | 1 | 2 | 3 | 4 | 5 | 6 | 7 | 8 | 9 | 10 | 11 | 12 | 13 | 14 | 15 | 16 | 17 | 18 | 19 | 20 | 21 | 22 | 23 | 24 | 25 | 26 | 27 | 28 | 29 | 30 | 31 |
|---|---|---|---|---|---|---|---|---|---|---|---|---|---|---|---|---|---|---|---|---|---|---|---|---|---|---|---|---|---|---|---|
| MISCELLANEOUS (continued) | | | | | | | | | | | | | | | | | | | | | | | | | | | | | | | |
| Resuscitation Forms | | | | | | | | | | | | | | | | | | | | | | | | | | | | | | | |
| Incident Reports | | | | | | | | | | | | | | | | | | | | | | | | | | | | | | | |
| Telephone number cards | | | | | | | | | | | | | | | | | | | | | | | | | | | | | | | |
| Medical Info. folder | | | | | | | | | | | | | | | | | | | | | | | | | | | | | | | |
| Cardiac Board | | | | | | | | | | | | | | | | | | | | | | | | | | | | | | | |
| Extension cord | | | | | | | | | | | | | | | | | | | | | | | | | | | | | | | |
| | | | | | | | | | | | | | | | | | | | | | | | | | | | | | | | |
| Initials: | | | | | | | | | | | | | | | | | | | | | | | | | | | | | | | |

# ADDENDUM E

## 8 West Unit Diagram

This diagram illustrates the physical layout of the nursing unit and the location of emergency equipment, exits, oxygen cutoff valves, fire alarms, and fire extinguishers. It also shows traffic flow and the break down of the three nursing teams: A, B, and C. It is used for orientation of new staff members.

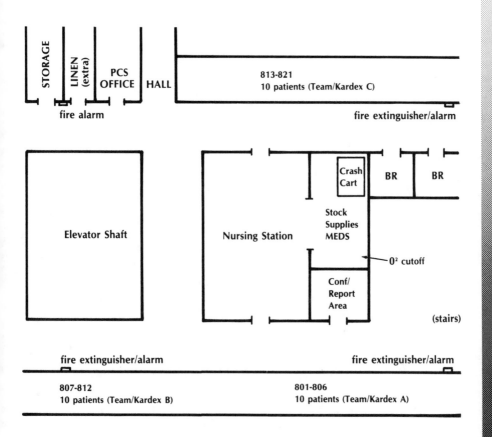

STORAGE

LINEN (extra)

PCS OFFICE

HALL

813-821
10 patients (Team/Kardex C)

fire alarm

fire extinguisher/alarm

Elevator Shaft

Nursing Station

Crash Cart

BR

BR

Stock Supplies MEDS

$O^2$ cutoff

Conf/ Report Area

(stairs)

fire extinguisher/alarm

fire extinguisher/alarm

807-812
10 patients (Team/Kardex B)

801-806
10 patients (Team/Kardex A)

# ADDENDUM F

## 8 West

## Staffing and Scheduling Policies

1. The usual staffing patterns for 8 West are:

   A. Weekdays:

      a. *Day shift* - preferred staff, 8; minimum staff, 6, at least 4 RN's; at least 4 out of 6 must be licensed and capable of administering medications.

      b. *Evening shift* - preferred staff, 5; minimum staff, 4, all of whom must be licensed and at least 3 of whom are RN's.

      c. *Night shift* - preferred staff, 4; minimum staffing 3, all of whom must be licensed and at least 2 of whom are RN's.

   B. Weekends:

      a. *Day shift* - preferred staff, 7; minimum staffing 6, at least 4 RN's; at least 4 out of 6 must be licensed and capable of administering medications.

      b. *Evening shift* - preferred staff, 4; minimum staffing 4, all of whom must be licensed and at least 3 of whom are RN's.

      c. *Night shift* - preferred staff, 3; minimum staffing 3, all of whom must be licensed and at least 2 of whom are RN's.

2. Scheduling is the overall responsibility of the PCS, with schedule-making delegated to a committee of four staff members, three full-time and one part-time, representing all three shifts. Schedules will cover a 4-week period. Supervised by the PCS, the committee will draw up the schedule during the first week of the 4-week period covered by the previous schedule and post the schedule during the third week of the previous schedule. All staff will eventually serve on this committee.

3. A request book is used to log preferred working schedules. Every effort will be made to honor reasonable requests for time off or preferred work times. However, these requests must be made before the midpoint of the posted schedule. Scheduling cycles will be regularly used and altered only on request or to accommodate vacations and holidays.

4. Vacations will be handled as outlined in Department of Nursing policy. Requests will be taken all year but must be submitted in most circumstances a minimum of 8 weeks in advance. As stated, staff are provided with two out of three weekends in a row off. If a third is desired, it must be arranged by the staff member.

5. Staff may make equal switches on the schedule ONLY AFTER a completed request change slip has been approved by a member of the staffing committee.

6. Cycle development is done in accordance with Department of Nursing policy.

Approval: 2/83
           PCS/ADN 8 West

Review: 2/87

Revision: 2/86

# ADDENDUM G

## Nursing Students on the Medical/Surgical Areas

Students from universities affiliated with the department of nursing may work on 8 West, with these limitations:

1. Nursing instructors will be responsible for establishing orientation dates for their students and for themselves. During the orientation, the instructors will meet with the PCS on the unit to learn the roles of various staff members, the physical layout, the unit charting procedures, and specific nursing care measures that their students will need to know. The students, during their orientation, will also meet with the PCS to review these matters, as well as fire and code responsibilities, assignment to a staff RN, and a review of the role of nursing students on a medical/surgical unit.

2. Nursing instructors are responsible for the actions of their students at all times. The nurses on 8 West function primarily as role models for students in providing daily care to the acutely ill patient. Both instructors and nurses will share responsibility for helping the students learn as much as they can at a pace that's comfortable for them and at a level compatible with their stage of preparation.

3. The nurses on 8 West reserve the right to interrupt or even stop students from performing nursing measures that may be harmful to the patients.

4. Nursing instructors will make student assignments the day before or the morning of a student's arrival on the unit.

5. The shift coordinator on the unit will assign an RN to each student as a "buddy".

6. Students will report to work at the designated shift time to attend report, receive their patient assignments, and accompany the RN's assigned to them on bedside rounds. The nursing instructor should attend the shift report to stay updated on the patient population and to identify possible learning opportunities for the students.

7. The nursing instructor will make early bedside rounds with the student/buddy groups to identify learning goals for the day. The staff must be informed of the students' needs in order to assist in their education.

8. Students may perform any nursing procedure that they have previously performed to standard. However, if the task is new or one which the student is not comfortable performing, then the nursing instructor must be present.

9. A grace period of one hour will be allowed for the administration of routine medications by the students. If a student feels she requires supervision, she should notify her nursing instructor. If the instructor can't observe during the one-hour grace period, the student buddy will give the medication.

10. Because they are not licensed, students may not:

    a. Administer I.V. medication;

    b. Instill additives (such as heparin or insulin) to main I.V. lines;

    c. Mix and hang emergency medical (such as lidocaine or dopamine);

    d. Initiate a Code. Students may notify the nursing staff of a life-threatening situation, however, and may begin CPR;

    e. Have keys to the narcotics cabinet in their possession. They may give oral narcotics obtained by the RN assigned to them;

    f. Take verbal orders from the doctor.

11. All students will be expected to provide nursing care on 8 West according to established standards. They must also document their nursing care, sign the patient's chart (and have either their buddy or instructor co-sign their nursing notes), and contribute to the care plan on the Kardex.

12. Students may hang routine I.V.s, administer piggyback I.V. medications, and start peripheral I.V. lines, if qualified, under the direct supervision of a staff member or their instructor.

13. Nurses should review procedures orally with students before letting students do them to validate that the student has the knowledge and skill needed to carry out the assignment.

APPROVED: JANUARY 1984
    PCS/ADN/DON
    Nursing staff 8 West
    Appropriate Instructor head

REVIEW: JANUARY 1987

REVISION: JANUARY 1986

## ADDENDUM H
### Delivery of Care Methodology for 8 West

1. The method of delivering patient care on 8 West can be described as the *case method* for total patient care.

   A. RN's provide total patient care for an assigned group of patients, working on a shift basis and with as much consistency as possible over days or weeks.

   B. Assignments of patients are generally based on the admitting RN, but may be distributed over the entire staff, if necessary. The assigned RN's will assume ongoing responsibility for updating care plans for their patients. Assignments will be closely coordinated, with care plans or primary responsibilities posted on the nursing station blackboard.

   C. Three teams of nurses—A, B, and C—will provide patient care over a 24-hour period. A "care planning RN" will serve as coordinator for each team. She will accomplish this task through oral instructions and through use of Kardex and shift report.

   D. Non-RN's will participate in the care of patients on 8 West, but the RN is accountable for the quality and effectiveness of that care. In addition:

   - The RN is responsible for determining the capabilities of nonprofessional staff members before delegating assignments.

   - The RN will perform the initial assessment on all newly admitted patients.

   E. Total patient care means carrying out all aspects of the nursing process, including assessment, nursing diagnosis, developing a care plan, performing those tasks that can't be delegated to nonprofessional staff, and evaluating the effectiveness of both medical and nursing interventions. It also implies the use of relevant standards (especially protocols and standards of care); medication administration; documentation (including physician orders); interaction with the doctor, shift coordinator, and the patient's family; and required discharge preparation and patient teaching.

   F. Shifts are normally eight hours long. Ten-hour shifts may be requested and integrated into the cycle, as necessary. Nursing responsibilities for times that overlap two shifts are explained in "Performance Standards for Extended Shifts".

2. Assignment:

   A. The shift coordinator will make assignments before each shift report to give the staff members an opportunity to focus on their patients during report. The assignments will be written on the unit assignment sheet and posted on the nursing station blackboard, where they can be referred to by the NOS and doctors.

B. Nurses will be assigned to patients on the basis of:

- patients needs,
- nurses' capabilities,
- availability of staff,
- staff learning needs,
- continuity of patient care,
- care planning assignments,
- physical layout of the unit,
- infection control measures.

C. Assignments may be changed during or after report, if necessary, by the shift coordinator or staff.

D. The care of all patients will be planned, directed, and evaluated by an RN, even though the care itself may be given to a non-RN.

E. Each nonprofessional staff member will be assigned to an RN whose name will appear beside hers on the assignment sheet. LPN's will assume a full patient-care load, with a backup RN available to carry out the nursing process and other professional responsibilities. Nursing assistants may be assigned to specific patients or RN's, or given functional assignments, as desired, by the shift team.

F. An RN will also be assigned to patients cared for by private-duty student nurses.

G. All staff members will fill out an assignment worksheet to organize their work and record their activities to prevent duplication of effort or the omission of important tasks.

3. Reports:

A. Shift reports will be taped about one hour before the end of each shift. These reports will focus on the status of each patient and significant medical and nursing interventions performed during the past shift. Routine medications, physician orders, and laboratory tests results will not be recorded, since this information can be found on the Kardex. (The oncoming shift is responsible for obtaining this information.)

B. Reports will cover patients by areas (A, B, and C), following this routine:

- the patient's name, age, doctor, and current diagnosis (with "no code" patients identified);
- status (preop, postop, diagnostic, and so forth);
- brief summary of the patient's condition during the previous shift including comfort, nutrition, mobility, intake and output, and cooperativeness;

- current status of I.V.'s and ongoing I.V. medications (other than routine);
- significant changes in medical or nursing care plans.

C. Standards of care, protocols in operation and patient's response as appropriate, on their assigned patients.

D. Immediately after report, all oncoming RN's and LPN's will talk with the nurses going off-duty to doublecheck information in the report, clarify points of confusion, and learn of any changes since the report was taped.

E. Walking rounds will be made for all Class III and IV patients to verify their conditions and the status of IV's, drains, tubes, and other equipment.

F. Oncoming nurses will review Kardexes to complete their assignment sheets. Each of the three sections on 8 West has a Kardex.

G. If walking rounds were not made with the offgoing staff, the oncoming nurses will then make rounds themselves to check each patient.

4. Shift Coordinator:

A. The PCS will assign an RN to be shift coordinator for each shift. A backup will also be assigned.

B. Addendum M lists specific roles and responsibilities of the shift coordinator. Generally, these include:

- assigning patients and unit duties, such as narcotics, stock drugs, and crash cart checks;

- coordinating the use of beds on the unit, the handling of emergency situations, and acknowledgement of physician orders during code blue situations;

- maintaining contact with the NOS, PCS, and ADN regarding unit problems and staffing;

- supervising and directing new staff members as well as all non-regular staff;

- solving problems that have to do with patient care, physician complaints, or interdepartmental conflicts;

- organizing education activities and care conferences, as planned by the PCS or the shift coordinator herself;

- classifying patients at the end of each shift using input from the staff;

- providing the PCS with a complete shift report and facilitating the nursing office report at end of each shift;

- attending weekly discharge planning rounds;

- taking patient assignments only when necessary and then only a minimum number with low acuity, to be available to the staff as much as possible.

5. LPN/NA Responsibilities:

A. LPN's will be expected to report to their designated RN at least three times per shift regarding:

- the status of patients assigned;
- progress with their workloads;
- validation of problem-solving actions;
- questions and concerns requiring professional direction.

B. NA's will be expected to report to their designated RN every 2 hours to review their workloads and possible changes of assignment.

APPROVAL: 3/84
         PCS/ADN 8 West
         DON
         Nursing staff 8 West

REVIEW: 3/87

REVISION: 3/86

# ADDENDUM I
## Staffing Policies for Medical/Surgical Areas

1. Selection of Staff:

   A. New staff members may be hired from outside the hospital or transferred from other areas. All applicants being considered for the 8 West staff will be interviewed by the PCS and ADN after their resumes are reviewed. The PCS will discuss the job description and performance standards with the applicant, emphasizing specific issues such as nursing responsibilities, scheduling, and the unit's participative style of management. Applicants will then take a tour of the unit.

   B. Every attempt will be made to hire nurses with previous medical/surgical experience compatible with 8 West's patient population. Applicants without such experience may still be considered if they show outstanding motivation or leadership potential.

   C. Generally, applicants must have at least one year of experience in medical/surgical nursing within the past three years. Otherwise, they will be referred to a refresher program. New graduates will be hired selectively to participate in the department of nursing and internship program on the unit. Refresher RN's will receive special consideration as outlined in departmental policy.

   D. Contingency staff, such as agent nurses, will not be used unless an extreme staffing shortage exists. In-house "float pools" will provide additional support staff. Contingency employees, such as nursing students, will be hired during peak summer vacation periods.

   E. Part-time nurses hired from outside the hospital will be expected to follow a full-time orientation schedule before beginning their part-time schedules. Specifically, part-time nurses will work dayshift for one week and rotation shift for another week before assuming their part-time schedule on an assigned shift.

   F. Regular part-time status requires at least four working days per pay period if the nurse is to maintain her nursing skills, contribute to unit projects, and stay abreast of changes on the unit.

2. Orientation:

   A. All newly-hired staff members on 8 West shall receive the general hospital and department of nursing orientation before assignment on the unit.

   B. New staff members will also be given a more specialized orientation to the unit standards for 8 West. This second orientation period will have written objectives and highly structured content. It will consist of a review of standards, a period of supervised patient care, and formal classes on 8 West's patient population. This orientation will last two weeks—one week on the 7 to 3 shift and a week of rotation to an alternate shift.

C. Being funded out of the unit's budget, this second orientation period is subject to change, depending on the patient population and staffing status. It may be extended another two weeks if the PCS or ADN feels that new staff members need the extra time to make a smooth transition to the unit.

3. Staff Preparation and Responsibility:

A. New staff members are expected to meet the minimum requirements for continued employment by the end of the three-month probationary period. These requirements include, but are not limited to, the following:

- demonstrates competence in basic assessment skills, care planning, nursing interventions, and application of the nursing process;

- demonstrates ability to communicate effectively with other nurses, doctors, supervisors, and patients and their families;

- demonstrates ability to document, in accordance with hospital, departmental, and unit standards;

- demonstrates knowledge of all unit policies, procedures, and written standards;

- demonstrates ability to serve as shift coordinator, which involves coordination, communication, and supervisory responsibilities.

B. New staff members will conduct self-evaluation during orientation to identify learning needs. They will collaborate with the PCS to avail themselves of unit and departmental learning activities that will help them meet these needs.

C. All staff members will attend critical care classes to meet specific learning needs.

D. All staff members will attend mandatory educational activities on 8 West and complete the basic learning modules on assessment, documentation, care planning, and the nursing process by the end of the probationary period.

E. All staff members will accept temporary reassignment to other units when necessary. For educational purposes, they will participate in planned rotation programs on other units.

4. Probationary Period:

A. New staff members will be evaluated by the PCS and ADN after the three-week hospital orientation period and the three-month probationary period. Between these two dates, the PCS and ADN will hold periodic conferences to discuss the progress of new staff members.

B. After evaluation of the probationary period, the staff member may be approved for continued employment. Goals for the rest of the year, including learning needs, will be set at this time.

C. PCS and ADN may decide to extend the probationary period for a staff member after notifying the coordinator of clinical education and personnel department.

D. Such an extension of the probationary period will be granted on an individual basis, with specific behavioral and performance goals set by the PCS and ADN and the staff member. Throughout the extension period, the staff member's progress must be closely documented.

E. At the end of the extension period, the PCS and ADN will decide whether the staff member should be retained for continued employment.

5. Staffing Changes and Requests:

A. Staff members must give at least four weeks notice before leaving their positions or requesting any change in status, such as a maternity leave, a leave of absence, or a change to part-time status.

B. A change to part-time status will be granted only after such a position becomes available and a suitable replacement is found for the staff member's full-time position.

C. All requests for a change from full-time to part-time status, or part-time to full-time status, or a change in the number of days worked per pay period, must be presented in writing by the staff member following discussion with the PCS. The request must be approved by the PCS and ADN and the personnel department. Once such a change has been approved, at least six months must elapse before another request for a change of status from the same staff member will be considered. Exceptions may be made for extenuating circumstances.

D. With regard to summer staffing schedules, note that a part-time employee may work full time during low staffing periods (if the staffing budget allows) and still maintain part-time status with PCS and ADN approval.

E. No request for schedule changes that would involve overtime will be granted unless requested or approved by the PCS, ADN, and NOS. For scheduling purposes, Saturday and Sunday constitute the weekend.

F. Regular part-time status requires at least four working days per pay period. This criterion will apply to all members requesting a change to such status.

6. Vacation Time:

   A. Nurses will be encouraged to use vacation time throughout the year to avoid staff shortages during the summer. Vacation requests should be submitted at least two months in advance to the PCS and scheduling committee. Retroactive vacation days will not be granted. The PCS may grant isolated vacation days if scheduling permits; these days should be requested at least two weeks in advance. If this isn't possible, the staff member may take the vacation day if she finds someone to replace her that day (See Addendum F).

   B. Isolated vacation days or holiday time may not be taken on a weekend when the staff member is scheduled to work unless she finds her own replacement.

   C. Staff members will be expected to work 26 out of 52 weekends. Vacation time will cover two consecutive weekends, one extra weekend for every week or vacation request. Every attempt will be made to schedule staff members so they have every other weekend off, but this policy may change during peak vacation periods. A staff member may only have a third weekend off, with two weeks vacation, if she finds her own replacement.

7. Leave of Absence:

   A. Leaves of absence will be granted only for those reasons stated in the hospital policy. Staffing needs may require that these positions be filled with regular staff members if temporary replacements can't be found.

   B. Consistent with personnel department and nursing policy, staff members on leaves of absence will be given first consideration for reemployment on the unit.

APPROVED: July, 1981
     PCS/ADN/DON 8 West
     Personnel Department
     Nursing Staff 8 West

REVIEW: July 1987

REVISION: July 1986

# RN STAFF NURSE PERFORMANCE STANDARDS —
## 8 WEST Medical-Surgical Unit

1. ASSESSMENT

   a. Performs admission assessment on all patients admitted within *24 hours* on NDB per guidelines.

   b. If initial admission on another unit, reviews this as baseline and completes unit assessment *within 20 minutes* after arrival of patient.

   c. Performs shift assessment *within 2 hours* of coming on duty to consist of:

   | | |
   |---|---|
   | NEURO: | LOC/mental status/orientation/psychological attitude |
   | CV: | Skin warmth/color, AR rate/respiration/BP, Neck veins @45. |
   | PUL: | Breathing patterns, Ant/post. chest sounds. |
   | GU/GI: | Abdominal flatness, softness, BS, flatus/BM; Urine qs/color/method. |
   | MS/INTEG: | ROM adequacy, Wound/dressing/tube condition/drainage, IV site/condition/infusion status, Skin condition (dependent areas for lesions/edema). |

   d. *Repeats shift assessment mid-point and end of shift* with focus on organ/system of pathology.

   e. Performs shift assessment at transfer or discharge from unit.

   f. Documents shift assessment on unit assessment flowsheet *within 2 hours* of coming on duty and *mid-point and end of shift* according to form guideline.

2. CARE PLANNING

   a. Pulls appropriate Standard of Care (SCP) and supportive protocols after admission assessment complete and in consideration of admission medical diagnosis (DRG). Implements these as outlined in "Guidelines for Use of Standards of Care and Protocols". Perform on all new admissions *within 8 hours after* arrival on unit.

   b. Retires completed protocols and adds new ones as needed.

   c. Activates nursing diagnosis and modifies/individualizes above *in writing* as specified in guidelines.

   d. Reviews each active nursing diagnosis *q 24 hours* for continuation of care, modification or discontinuation as specified in guidelines.

   e. Adds to standard of care as necessary according to guidelines.

f. Uses blank kardex NCP for additional nursing management not addressed via standards:

    (1) specify nursing diagnosis (from approved list);
    (2) specify patient outcome;
    (3) specify independent and dependent nursing measures.

g. Integrates nursing plan of care with medical plan of care.

3. EVALUATION

a. Performs ongoing evaluation of effectiveness *each shift* as indicated by shift assessment and appropriate alteration of care.

b. Enters either evaluation or resolution date on SCP *each day shift of duty.*

c. Judges the effectiveness of current protocols on patient *each shift.*

d. Judges the effectiveness of current standards of care on patient *each shift.*

e. Judges the effectiveness of each medication administered to patient *each shift.*

f. Judges the effectiveness of comfort measures including all PRN meds given *within 1 hour of intervention.*

g. Evaluates patient response to all procedures carried out both on a physical and psychological basis.

h. Judges patients psychological response to hospitalization and diagnosis each shift.

i. Evaluates patient's/SO's self care responsibilities in relation to teaching protocols carried out.

j. Evaluates effectiveness of all medical treatments administered on a shift basis including but not limited to:
- IV therapy,
- wound/dressing care,
- blood product administration,
- alternate feeding measures.

4. TECHNICAL SKILLS

A. Performs following skills as outlined in nursing procedures:
- Start/DC peripheral IV;
- Insert/DC NG/sumps/feeding tubes/irrigation of same;
- Change establish trachs;
- Insert naso-pharyngeal airways;
- Aspirate blood from CVP lines;

- Suction all airways (mouth, nose, trach, mushroom/trumpets);
- Insert/irrigate/DC M/F foleys;
- Set-up bedframe/trapeze;
- Irrigate ostomy wounds.

b. Assists physicians with the following measures:

- CVP insertion,
- cutdown,
- spinal tap,
- bedside bronchoscopy,
- bedside thoracentesis/paracentesis,
- CT insertion,
- Declotting of AV shunts,
- Complex dressing changes,
- Hickman line insertion.

c. Uses equipment according to nursing procedures:

- IV controller/pumper,
- Gomco,
- Pleurevac,
- hypothermia blanket,
- Wall suction,
- Patient bed (all 6 positions),
- Crash cart,
- Ambu bag,
- CPM device,
- Patient roller,
- Century bath,
- circo-electric bed,
- stryker frame,
- air mattress,
- kinetic bed,
- K-pad,
- blood warmer,
- Volumetric pump,
- Trach trays,
- Cutdown trays,
- Blood pump,
- Geri-chair,
- Cardiac monitor (emergency basic attachment only).

5. PATIENT EDUCATION

a. Assesses patient's learning needs and performs following *teaching protocols:*

- Diabetic teaching protocol,
- Pre-op teaching protocol,
- Colostomy teaching protocol,
- Hickman line teaching protocol.

b. Evaluates patient's response to above protocols in areas specified in protocol; documents as specified.

6. DOCUMENTATION

a. Completes the following Department and unit tools according to established guidelines:

- Nursing Data Base,
- Nursing Flowsheet (for standards)
- Nursing Progress Record,
- I/O sheet,
- Medication record,
- Graphic record,
- Frequent V/S sheet,
- Crashcart checklist,
- Unit assignment,
- Individual worksheet,
- Narcotics records,
- Code Blue forms,
- Incident reports,
- Assessment flowsheet.

b. Cosigns MD orders by end of shift and stats within 10 minutes of written orders.

c. Opens charts with assessment flowsheet by midshift.

d. Charts NPR summation prior to end of shift with focus on:
    1.) Symptomatology noted, intervention, evaluation of effectiveness,
    2.) Change from baseline assessment,
    3.) Evaluation statement on protocols in effect,
    4.) Evaluation statement on standards of care in effect.

e. Uses only hospital approved abbreviations.

f. Writes legibly at all times.

g. Records verbal orders only in the following circumstances:
    1.) Emergency situations,
    2.) Code Blue activities,
    3.) Rapid transfers.

h. Places verbal orders on physician order sheet within 20 minutes of taking them and only during tour of duty.

i. Follows all Department of Nursing generic performance standards for documentation with reference to (including but not limited to):
    1.) signatures/titles,
    2.) no blanks,
    3.) error correction,
    4.) Blue/blank ink only,
    5.) Addressograph on all front back and single sheets.

j. Charts implementation of each protocol and standard of care in effect on Standards NFS, entering and discontinuing as specified in form guidelines.

k. Correctly completes chart forms for diagnostic work:
    1.) Lab,
    2.) xray,
    3.) Nuclear medicine,
    4.) EKG/ECHO.

7. PATIENT RIGHTS / LEGAL ISSUES

a. Adheres to *system requirements* in the following areas of *Structure:*

1.) Patient confidentiality of information,
2.) Use of media (news, radio, TV) requests,
3.) Regulations governing staff as witness to legal actions,
4.) Knowledge of Hospital Patient Bill of Rights,
5.) Regulations governing patient's access to chart.

b. Protects patient's privacy (physical and psychological).

c. Meets patient's right to be informed.

d. Protects patient's valuables as specified by hospital policy.

8. SAFETY

a. Completes incident reports with:

1) all patient unusual incidents (order transcription, etc),
2) Patient/SO falls,
3) Medication/IV errors,
4) SO complaints,
5) SO/visitor/employee injury,
6) Lost equipment/belongings,
7) Inaccurate narcotic count,
8) All reports of events to security (traffic control violations, suspicious persons, etc),
9) Physician complaints.

b. Adheres to all unit/Department safety policies:

1) Infection control,
2) Restraints,
3) Fire reporting/drill activities,
4) Disaster reporting/drill activities,
5) Electrical safety policies,
6) Transport safety policies,
7) Safety policies for risk prevention in Dependent patients,
8) Traffic control/visitor policies,
9) Equipment maintenance.

9. EMERGENCY SITUATIONS

a. Responds to the following unit/patient crisis situations as outlined in protocols for nursing:

1) Hypovolemic shock,
2) Rapid IV cannulation,
3) CPR,
4) Respiratory crisis (obstruction, apnea, aspiration),
5) Loss of orthopedic tissue perfusion (with casts, traction),
6) Loss of AV shunt integrity,
7) Neurologic complications (seizures, decreased LOC),

8) Acute pulmonary edema,
9) Tension pneumothorax,
10) Hypoglycemia.

b. Documents events and patients response as well as intervention as specified in above protocols.

10. KNOWLEDGE BASE

a. Maintains working knowledge of unit level Structure standards/policies for operation of this nursing unit in the following areas:

1) Description of unit;
2) Purpose of nursing unit;
3) Objectives of nursing unit;
4) Administration of and organization of nursing unit including the organizational chart, narrative, and verbage detailing medical and nursing responsibilities;
5) Hours of operation;
6) Utilization of the nursing unit including admission; duration of stay, discharge criteria/planning policies;
7) Governing rules of the nursing unit including all previously mentioned safety/physical environment issues;
8) Staffing policies including:
   • quantity requirements,
   • levels of workers,
   • preparation requirements,
   • credentialing requirements;
9) Nursing responsibilities that are allowed and supported to be carried out on this unit.

b. Maintains working knowledge of Department of Nursing Structure standards/policies for operation of the Department of Nursing as outlined in the Generic DON Standards Manual.

c. *Locates and uses the unit and Department of Nursing Standards Manuals.*

d. Locates and uses the *unit files* for implementation of protocols and standards of care as specified in guidelines for use.

e. Locates and uses other *reference manuals* and books on the nursing unit:

1) Personnel manual,
2) Dietary manual,
3) Lab manual,
4) Nuclear medicine manual,
5) Pharmacy manual,
6) Ancellary services manual,
7) Hospital administration Policy manual,

8) Unit library,

9) Department of Nursing/Hospital library.

f. Performs *essential unit protocols:*,

1) Chest tube,
2) IV therapy,
3) GU intubation,
4) GI intubation,
5) Blood products transfusion,
6) Pre-op,
7) Post-op,
8) Restraint,
9) Skin integrity,
10) Immobility,
11) Pain,
12) Coma,
13) AV shunt,
14) Traction/cast/CPM,
15) Insulin,
16) TPN,
17) Tube feeding,
18) Lipid infusion,
19) Depression,
20) Anticoagulation,
21) Hypothermia,
22) Basic monitoring parameters/physical hygiene,
23) Artificial airway.

g. Manages patients on the following high risk or titrated *medications:*

1) Digitalis,
2) Lasix,
3) NTG (long acting PO, paste, and SL),
4) IV narcotics,
5) Multiple antibiotics,
6) CNS depressants (barbiturates, tranquilizers of thorazine, valium, phenobarb).

# PROCEDURE

# HOSPITAL
## DEPARTMENT OF NURSING
### CHEST TUBE INSERTION/DRAINAGE PROCEDURE

*PURPOSE:* To outline the nursing responsibilities in assisting the physician with insertion of a closed system drainage chest tube.

*SUPPORTIVE DATA:* Chest tubes are used to evacuate accumulated air, blood, pus or fluid from the thoracic cavity, to reestablish negative pressure in the intrapleural space, and thereby explain the lung/s following collapse resulting from surgery or trauma. The system is a closed drainage one and may consist of a combination disposable device or glass bottles of the non-disposable type (water-seal, water-seal and suction, or water-seal, suction, and drainage). Tubes are usually placed in the second intercostal space anteriorly to remove air and the eighth or ninth intercostal space posteriorly to remove fluid. Only physicians are allowed to insert, irrigate, and remove chest tubes. Licensed staff may assist with insertion.

*EQUIPMENT LIST:* (from CSR and clean unit treatment room)

- Thoracentesis tray (containing 1% plain xylocaine; sterile connectors both straight and Y type; betadine swabs, 2 pair size 7½ gloves; needles; silk suture; needle holder; straight kelly clamp; tissue forceps; thoracic catheters (32 Fr., 28 Fr., 20 Fr.) 1 set trocars; knife handle and blades)
- Plastic disposable chest drainage system
- 2" adhesive Tape,
- Betadine ointment,
- Wall suction gauge and connecting tubing,
- Sterile water (500cc) & 50cc toumy tip syringe,
- 2 medium Kelly clamps from CSR (rubber shod)

*CONTENT:*

| STEPS | KEY POINTS |
|---|---|
| 1. Prepare patient for procedure by explanation and assuring permit is signed. | |
| 2. Assemble equipment and take to bedside. Follow directions on chest drainage system. Keep all connections sterile. | • Take a few minutes to review the equipment, tracing the suction and drainage. |

# SUCTION CHAMBER

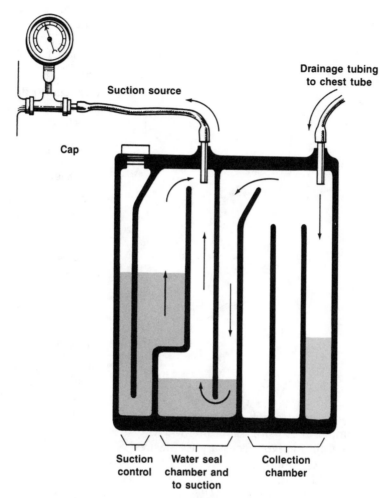

a. Attach sterile 50 ml. irrigation syringe, without barrel, to rubber tubing of water seal chamber.

b. Fill water seal chamber to 2 cm line.

• Even though water will not come into contact with patient, it should be sterile.

• Water seal chamber must be filled *first* and maintained at 2 cm to create a seal for closed drainage; this is filled regardless of whether suction is applied from wall.

- If patient to be on straight drainage, cap may be left off; otherwise reapply to reduce or muffle suction bubbling noise.

- Physician orders amount of suction, usually 20 cm.

- Keep in plain view to prevent accidental breakage.

- Excessive bubbling is not necessary; amount of chest suction is controlled by water level not wall gauge.

- Too much bubbling creates noise and rapid evaporation of water level.

- Main complete sterility of field until tube is in and connected to drainage.

c. Remove cap from suction control chamber and, using same method as above, fill to level necessary for desired amount of suction. Replace cap. *DO NOT OBSTRUCT AIR VENT TO ALLOW ESCAPE OF AIR FROM PATIENT.*

d. Hang unit from bed or place in support devices.

e. Connect suction tubing to wall suction and adjust gauge to produce *slight continuous bubbling* in suction chamber.

3. Open thoracostomy tray; assist with setting up sterile field; provide trash receptacle to keep field organized; assist physician as necessary; assist patient to remain calm, comfortable, and motionless as possible.

4. When tube is in, hand physician sterile end of drainage connecting tubing so it can be attached to the 5:1 sterile connector.

5. Secure all connections at the patient end and wall suction end with spiraling adhesive tape. *Always use adhesive tape and leave area at connector where drainage is visible.*

6. Assist physician with dressing using betadine ointment, several 4 × 4's, large ABD, and adhesive tape. Elastoplast is also excellent. When dressing is complete, attach a final piece of adhesive tape in a split-tape (vertical) to dressing and chest tube in a spiral fashion.

   - Provide secure, supportive dressing; do not use paper tape.

   - This secures tube and prevents excessive pull on tubing from bed clothes and equipment.

7. Position patient for comfort. Implement "Chest Tube Protocol" for ongoing care.

8. Return equipment to CSR after rinsing.

9. Document procedure including patient's tolerance and any difficulties during insertion in NPR.

   - Place rubber-shod Kelly clamps at the head of the bed with tape in plain view.

## CHANGING DRAINAGE DEVICE

A licensed nurse may change the drainage device when it is damaged or reaches 2400 cc.

1. Set up new system with water seal and suction chambers filled to proper levels with sterile water.

   - Follow above steps.

   - Reverse clamps—one in one direction and the other opposite.

2. Explain activity to patient as appropriate.

3. Double clamp chest tube(s) close to insertion site. *Turn suction at wall to very low.*

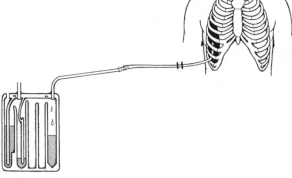

4. Remove old tape from upper end of connector; disconnect old drainage tubing and reconnect new tubing complete with new 5:1 connector. Tape as outlined.

5. Remove chest tube clamps and return suction wall gauge to produce slight constant bubbling in suction chamber.

- Turning down suction when changing system prevents pulmonary tissue trauma when clamps are removed.

6. Observe for constant suction chamber bubbling; observe for air leak in suction chamber; if excessive, follow protocol check.

7. Document system change and any difficulties in NPR.

## SPECIMEN COLLECTION

*A licensed nurse may collect specimen drainage as ordered by the physician.*

1. Clean specimen port on back of collection chambers with alcohol.

- Diaphragm is self sealing.

2. Use 18-20 gauge needle/syringe to withdraw sample.

3. Label syringe and send to lab with proper slip.

- Never use this method to attempt to empty the drainage device.

## DISCONTINUING THE CHEST TUBE

A licensed nurse may assist with discontinuing a chest tube when chest xrays have established the lung to be re-expanded.

Equipment:
- sterile gloves
- clamps from head board
- vaseline gauze
- suture removal pack
- 3 4x4's
- 2 or 3 inch adhesive tape

1. Explain procedure to patient.

2. Place patient in semi-Fowlers position.

3. Prepare materials by opening packs and placing vaseline gauze on top of stacked 4x4's. Have clamps present.

4. Physician will clamp tubes or ask you to do so; he will place the dressing over the insertion site, instruct patient to take a deep breath and hold it, and quickly remove the tube.

5. Secure dressing with adhesive tape.

- Protect bed with pad. Dressing must be ready to apply to insertion site prior to tube removal so vaseline gauze creates a seal to prevent sucking air leak.

- Tape promptly and securely, making sure vaseline gauze is against skin.

6. Document events and patient's tolerance in NPR.

- Physician may close wound with purse string suture.

REFERENCES: Bricker, Patricia Lee, Chest Tubes, RN November, 1980 American Journal of Nursing, How to Work with Chest Tubes (Programmed Instruction), 1980

APPROVAL:

REVIEW:

REVISION:

DISTRIBUTION:

# PROTOCOL

P
R
O
C
E
S
S

P
R
O
T
O
C
O
L
S

# HOSPITAL
## DEPARTMENT OF NURSING

| | INITIATED | DISCONTINUED |
|---|---|---|
| *CHEST TUBE/* | DATE _____ | DATE _____ |
| *CLOSED DRAINAGE* | TIME _____ | TIME _____ |
| *SYSTEM PROTOCOL* | RN _____ | RN _____ |

*PURPOSE:* To outline the nursing management of patients with one or more chest tubes connected to disposable closed drainage system.

*LEVEL:* Independent (requires nursing order only).

*CONTENT:*

*ASSESSMENT*

1. Assess the following parameters on initial insertion/admission and q̄ 2 hours:
   ▲ Observe breathing pattern, rate, symmetry
   ▲ Auscultate quality of breath sounds on both affected and unaffected sides
   ▲ Observe wound/chest tubes for:
     • bleeding, character of drainage
     • SQ emphysema
     • pressure dressing intact
   ▲ Observe chest tubes/drainage system:
     • all tubings unkinked/unobstructed and draining freely

     • all connections secured and taped with adhesive

     • free fluctuation in chest tube and water seal chamber

     • P/A air leak from patient evidenced by bubbling in water seal chamber

     • 2 cm water seal level

     • 15-20 cm water in suction chamber with low constant bubbling

     • chest tubes labeled according to physician op note

     • amount of drainage increase after each stripping; amount of drainage increase q̄ 2 hours × 48; then q̄ 4

## REPORTABLE CONDITIONS

2. Report the following conditions to the physician (who inserted chest tube) immediately:

▲ new or accelerating SQE

▲ deterioration in v/s or any indication of clogged tubes, respiratory distress, hypovolemic shock, or excessive water seal air leak

▲ bleeding in excess of 100cc/hour × 2 hours or more than 450cc/shift

▲ any irregularity in function of drainage system

## POSITION/CHEST CARE

3. ▲ Place patients in semi-fowlers 30-45 degrees (position of comfort)

▲ Turn & position all patients q̄ 2 hours from side to side, avoiding back for more than 1 hour; patients are to be propped and fully supported for comfort to promote optimum positions for breathing and drainage.

▲ Use rolled towels to prevent patient from lying on and kinking chest tubes (when on affected side)

▲ Cough & deep breath all patients q̄ 2 hours; pillows are to be used to splint the wound during treatments; chest P.T. (light cupping and vibration on exhalation) to be administered to posterior and lateral bilateral chest wall q̄ 4 hours until tube discontinued; collaborate with physician if endotrachial suctioning required (unless patient has artificial airway).

▲ Perform ROM to affected arm and shoulder 2× per shift.

▲ Keep drainage system below patient level at all times.

▲ Use two (2) staff members to get patient OOB with bed wheels in locked position at all times and to ambulate patient (when ordered by MD).

## CHEST TUBE CARE

4. Strip chest tubes on all patients.

q̄ 15 minutes × 4 (hour #1)
q̄ 30 minutes × 4 (hours #2, 3)
q̄ hour × 3 (hours #4, 5, 6)

q̄ 2 hours × 24 hours

q̄ 4 hours thereafter until drainage stops and lung is re-expanded

5. Utilize strippers or K-Y hand method

6. Add water to the suction chamber when evaporation takes it below the ordered suction level.

7. **Never** routinely clamp chest tubes but keep rubber shod large Kelly clamps (2) secured to head board at all times.

8. Maintain all patients on q̄ 8 hour I/O with drainage system marked a minium of q̄ hour × 8 hours and then each shift.

9. Maintain all tubings straight along bed edge and coiled for proper drainage (secure with rubber band and safety pin). *DO NOT ALLOW TUBING TO LOOP BELOW PATIENT EITHER IN BED OR CHAIR OR WHEN AMBULATING.*

## PAIN MANAGEMENT

10. Question all patients about pain q̄ 2 hours unless obviously asleep and medicate a minimum of q̄ shift × 48 hours. Sedate patients at a level of comfort to allow them to carry out necessary treatments.

## BEDSIDE SUPPLIES

11. Keep at the bedside at all times:

- extra sterile drainage system
- sterile straight and Y connector
- K-Y jelly packs
- betadine swabs
- 1 and 2 inch adhesive

- vaseline—gauze
- stripper
- 2 rubber-shod clamps
- abdominal dressing

## MD Communication

12. Collaborate daily with MD on:
- need for chest xray
- activity level progression
- anticipated discontinuation of tube

## DOCUMENTATION

13. ▲ Document the implementation of the protocol on the Standards flowsheet each shift.

▲ Enter an evaluative statement in the shift summary note in the NPR to indicate patient and system status and effectiveness of chest tube in maintaining effective ventilation; also document character of chest tube drainage on shift assessment flowsheet; maintain I & O record each shift on I & O Record.

*SAFETY*

14. Restrain upper extremeties for safety of any patient with altered LOC or any signs of confusion.

*EMERGENCY MEASURES*

15. CONTAINER AT CAPACITY: Change the drainage device at 2400 cc capacity. Document in NPR.

16. DISCONNECT: If chest tube becomes disconnected, the tube is to be immediately clamped (double) as close to the patient as possible. Both exposed ends are to be cleaned with betadine swabs for 30 seconds and left to air dry for 30 seconds. The drainage system is then to be re-connected using fresh adhesive tape. The RN is to remain at the patient's side during this time, assessing for respiratory distress which indicates suction must be re-established immediately.

Once suction/water seal re-established, a full chest assessment is to be done. Incident will be reported to the physician and discussion about possible chest xray should take place.

*Note:* If tube connections have been grossly contaminated, such as with urine, feces, etc., a new drainage system including sterile connector must be attached. If this option is carried out, it must be done swiftly (3-5 minutes) to prevent respiratory distress due to possible tension pneumothorax.

Document events, intervention, and patient response in NPR.

17. DISLODGEMENT: If tube is accidentally pulled out, promptly apply vaseline gauze and several 4 × 4's; page MD stat; prepare for new tube insertion; *do not tape—hold until help arrives;* stay with patient; observe for respiratory distress which may occur from tension pneumothorax; if dyspnea occurs, remove dressing and pressure for several minutes to allow air to escape and replace dressing; alternate this approach every 5 minutes until physician arrives.

18. TENSION PNEUMOTHORAX: Observe for acute respiratory distress characterized by increased respiratory rate, shallow respirations, cyanosis, decreased breath sounds, asymetrical breathing, failure of chest tube and/or water seal chamber to fluctuate or bubble. Notify physician stat;

check all connections for air leak; strip tube(s) in attempt to dislodge blockage; prepare for new tube insertion; obtain stat chest xray if ordered by MD; stay with patient; place in high fowlers; start oxygen at 4L/minute via cannula; monitor V/S q̄ 5 minutes; monitor for arrhythmias; prepare for ABG's determination as ordered by MD.

19. ☐ EXCESSIVE AIR LEAK: ☐ If water seal chamber bubbling continuously and excessively, check patient and system for air leak.

▲ Clamp chest tube close to chest wall; if bubbling stops, then air leak inside; notify MD immediately.

▲ If bubbling continues, unclamp tubes and apply pressure using both hands around insertion site as air may be entering chest around wound; if bubbling diminishes with pressure, notify MD and discuss replacing dressing with another pressure dressing. A suture may be required around tube.

▲ If neither measure decreases bubbling, air leak may be in tubing and or connections; secure all connections and retape. Tubing may be clamped at lower levels to locate specific leak; if retaping does not correct problem, change system.

*REFERENCES:*
*APPROVAL:*
*REVIEW/REVISION:*
*DISTRIBUTION:*

**HOSPITAL**
**DEPARTMENT OF NURSING**

| INITIATED | DISCONTINUED |
|---|---|
| DATE _____ | DATE _____ |
| TIME _____ | TIME _____ |
| RN _____ | RN _____ |

TEACHING PROTOCOL
FOR: *NEW COLOSTOMY PATIENT*

PURPOSE: To outline nursing responsibility in patient education of a patient/SO with a new colostomy.

LEVEL:    Independent (requires nursing order only)

CONTENT:

| OUTCOME STANDARDS: | DATE MET/SIGN |
|---|---|
| PHYSIOLOGIC: ▶ The colostomy patient will achieve and maintain normal bowel function through effective self care. | |
| PYSCHOLOGIC: ▶ The colostomy patient will demonstrate an attitude of acceptance of modified life style (altered bowel function and body image). | |
| COGNITIVE: ▶ The colostomy patient will demonstrate the ability to manage his colostomy independently (or with SO assistance). | |

| Information to be delivered | Methodology | Taught by/date | Patient/SO Response |
|---|---|---|---|
| *BAG* | | | |
| 1. Teach patient to apply/change colostomy bag using home device and equipment. | • Follow procedure for bag application/change<br>• Demonstrate on model<br>• Return demo by patient with assistance × 2<br>• Return demo by patient independently × 1 | | |
| 2. Review how to recognize when bag needs changing | • Explain/use booklet pictures to define:<br> ▲ release of flatus by opening end<br> ▲ after evacuation (with odor or weight to disturb seal) | | |
| *SKIN* | | | |
| 3. Teach proper skin and stoma care | • Stress importance of gentle daily/PRN cleansing with soap/water<br>• Review use of acetone/betadine on skin<br>• Demonstrate use of karaya ring<br>• Review s/s of skin/stoma irritation: redness, itching, pain, bleeding, excoriation<br>• Review use of karaya powder and seeing MD/RN if no improvement in 48 hours. | | |

## TEACHING PROTOCOL
### FOR: *NEW COLOSTOMY PATIENT (continued)*

| Information to be delivered | Methodology | Taught by/date | Patient/SO Response |
|---|---|---|---|
| **EQUIPMENT** | | | |
| 4. Teach cleaning and care of equipment | • Demon. and return demo. cleaning of bag and equipment with soap/water and proper hanging to dry × 1 | | |
| **IRRIGATION** | | | |
| 5. Teach how to irrigate colostomy on regular basis for maximum control and physiologic bowel function | • Follow procedure on colostomy irrigation; | | |
| | • Demonstrate on model | | |
| | • Return demo. by patient with assistance × 2 | | |
| | • Return demo. by patient independently | | |
| | • Discuss past BM habits and devise time schedule with patient based on his needs | | |
| | • Review measures to control odor (drops, tablets, bag rinsing) | | |
| **DIET** | | | |
| 6. Teach dietary regulation for best functioning of colostomy | • Have dietition see patient/SO for diet instruction to maintain stool consistency, reduce flatus, constipation, diarrhea | | |
| | • Review possible measures for diarrhea and constipation; instruct pt. to seek MD/RN attention if ineffective | | |
| **SUPPORT** | | | |
| 7. Generate frequence discussions with patient/SO focusing on his ability to lead a productive life; attempt to illicit his feelings about modified life style and altered body image. | • Provide and discuss booklet on "Living with a Colostomy". | | |
| | • Provide info on local clubs and arrange meeting with community representative if patient desires. | | |

## TEACHING PROTOCOL
### FOR: *NEW COLOSTOMY PATIENT* (continued)

| Information to be delivered | Methodology | Taught by/date | Patient/SO Response |
|---|---|---|---|
| *DOCUMENTATION* | | | |
| 8. Document all teaching activities in appropriate columns provided on this form as well as patient/helper response. Use additional progress notes below to add further explanation about patient's level of understanding and ability for self care. 9. Add date and signature to indicate patient's accomplishment of the outcome standards on front of protocol. | | | |

NURSING PROGRESS RECORD: (Use to summarize any pertinent nursing remarks needed to supplement above general comments about patient's and family's self care activity.)

| Date | Entry | Signature/Title |
|---|---|---|
| | | |

REFERENCES:
APPROVAL:
REVIEW:
REVISION:
DISTRIBUTION:

# HOSPITAL
## DEPARTMENT OF NURSING

*HYPOGLYCEMIA*
*PROTOCOL*

*PURPOSE:* To outline nursing responsibilities and management of a known diabetic patient experiencing acute signs and symptoms of hypoglycemia.

*LEVEL:* Dependent (requires physician's order on admission)

*SUPPORTIVE DATA:* Acute hypoglycemia is a medical emergency usually seen in unstable insulin dependent diabetics as well as stable diabetics whose medical regimen or usual routine is altered (ie. altered eating or activity schedules, other system illness, change from long-acting insulin to sliding scale, and so forth.) Blood sugars <45mg% for significant periods of time contribute to loss of consciousness, seizure activity, and possibly brain damage and must be corrected immediately.

*CONTENT:*

1. If patient is assessed to be *non-responsive* to verbal or non-verbal stimuli, perform the following:

   • Assess ventilation and cardiac status; if inadequate, begin CPR as indicated.

   • If ventilation and cardiac status adequate, assess neurologic status (pupillary response and response to noxious stimuli), if pupils still reactive and non-dilated, place in supine position with hyperextension of neck/jaw; insert plastic airway if no gag reflex present; suction as required.

   • Peform dextrostick—if results <45, administer 50 cc 50% glucose direct IV push or via existing IV

   • Notify MD stat

   • Draw stat blood sugar immediately out of opposite arm. Try to do this simultaneously (with assistance) as detrostick is being obtained.

   • If patient not immediately responsive, start IV of 500 cc D5W with 18 g. needle or catheter and infuse at 100cc per hour.

   • Document all activities in Nurses Progress Records, Intake and Output sheets, and medication records.

   • Stay with patient and begin routine assessments q̄ 15 minutes until physician arrives.

- Institute safety precautions of side rails and low bed position until appropriate level of consciousness demonstrated in patient.

2. If patient is assessed to be *awake but has a GCS <15,* perform the following:

   - Perform dextrostick; if results <45, administer 50 cc 50% glucose IV as above.

   - If >45, and swallowing/gag reflex adequate, administer 8 oz. orange juice with 2 packs sugar.

   - If >45, and aspiration is likely due to deficient gag/swallowing reflex or LOC, administer IV glucose as above.

   - If level of consciousness does not immediately improve, start IV as above.

   - Notify MD stat

   - Draw stat blood sugar (as above, try to do so as soon as possible for accurate reflection of blood sugar status responsible for symptoms)

   - Document protocol on Standards Flowsheet; record effectiveness of intervention on NPR.

*REFERENCE:*
*APPROVAL:*
*REVIEW:*
*REVISION:*
*DISTRIBUTION:*

# HOSPITAL
## DEPARTMENT OF NURSING

| INITIATED | DISCONTINUED |
| --- | --- |
| DATE _____ | DATE _____ |
| TIME _____ | TIME _____ |
| RN _____ | RN _____ |

*RESPIRATORY*
*PROTOCOL*

*PURPOSE:* To outline the nursing management of respiratory status in the care of artificial airways.

*LEVEL:* Interdependent (requires physician's order for dependent functions*)

*CONTENT:*

### Trach Care & ET Tube Care

1. Perform trach care q̄ 8 hours, minimum, with cleansing of the inner cannual per procedure (peroxide soak with water rinse). Clean site with peroxide and bedadine and apply new dressing. Change tapes q̄od and PRN. (All dressings will be precut or folded, not cut 4×4's.) Chart wound condition each shift on the Assessment Flow Sheet.

2. Provide all artificial airway care under sterile conditions with thorough handwashing before and after.

3. Provide all artificial airway patients with constant call bell/tap bell and magic slate for communication.

### Wrist Restraints

4. Restrain all intubated patients with hospital approved wrist restraints at all times except when under direct care or observation by a licensed nurse or paralyzed pharmacologically. Maintain appropriate circulation and exercise 2× per shift.

### Cuffs

5. Validate that cuffs of all tubes are low pressure/soft flabby type to minimize barotrauma to the trachea. (The only exception shall be short term post op patients from the OR.)

6. Keep cuffs inflated to protect airway from aspiration and establish seal for ventilation. Only the amount of air necessary to achieve a minimal leak (MLT) shall be used. To do this, air is injected into the cuff while positive pressure is exerted on the patients airway by ventilator or bag until no air leak is heard over the trachea or felt

over the mouth or nose; then ½ to 1 cc is removed. If patient on PEEP, maintain NLT (do not remove air.)

*Cuff Pressure*

7. Perform pressure readings and record at the beginning of each shift, using the pressure gauge with pressure maintained at less than 25 mm.

*Cuff Deflation*

8. Deflate cuffs on intubated patients (ET and trach) at least once each shift, for the purpose of removing pooled secretions accumulated above the cuff.

   a. Suction nasopharynx (mouth and nose) prior to deflation.
   b. Apply positive pressure bagging to the airway on inspiration during cuff deflation to force secretions up into mouth for suctioning.
   c. Omit this activity if patient on PEEP.
   d. Other routine cuff deflation is not necessary.

9. Secure all ET tubes with double-back, 2-inch adhesive tape in head halter fashion to be changed every shift and PRN. Use benzoin to protect skin from irritation.

10. Maintain plastic airways in place on patients with ET tubes if patients are agitated and/or bite the tube; otherwise it is not necessary.

*Oral Hygiene*

11. Provide mouth care (and appropriate nose care) q̄ 4 hours; change oral airway at this time; move oral ET tube alternately from side to side of mouth.

12. Insure that all artificial airway patients receive humidified air/$O_2$.

*Suctioning*

13. Suction PRN as indicated by chest sounds accompanied by hyperinflation and hyperoxygenation before, between, and after suction attempts; limit to 10 seconds; observe for arrhythmias.

14. Insure that patients on blow-by have cuffs inflated at all times unless otherwise ordered to reduce airway resistance and prevent aspiration.

*Cultures*

    * 15. Obtain sputum cultures, not to include sensitivity, initially on all patients with trachs and ET tubes; Repeat cultures on consultation with physician.

*Xrays*

    * 16. Obtain portable chest xrays routinely on all patients after intubation unless ordered otherwise. After correct placement is ascertained, mark the tube with marker or tape at the entrance to the patient's mouth. No more than 2-3 inches should extend from the patient's mouth/nose. Cut off excess to prevent kinking.

    17. Insure that patients who are sedated or have decreased LOC or who cannot/will not deep breath on command are ambued during chest xray (assistant to wear lead apron).

*Bedside Equipment*

    18. Keep the following equipment at bedside at all times:

- Extra sterile trach/ET tube of same size
- Complete suction set up (catheters ½ size tube diameter)
- Tonsil tip suction for mouth suction
- 2 syringes (one for use and one for backup for cuff inflation)
- Small rubber-shod clamp (in case of leaky cuff seal)
- Manual resuscitation bag
- Double oxygen hook-up (one for ventilator; one for bag)
- Spirometer

*Tube Changes*

    19. Validate that in patients with oral ET tubes, communication with the physician take place after 24 hours about the possibility of nasal re-entubation for ease of care and patient comfort.

    20. There is no established time period for changing nasal ET tubes or trachs. Discuss with physician if tube seems clogged or difficult to keep clear.

    * 21. RN staff in Critical Care Areas (ICU/CCU) may change a trach which is established (longer than 24 hours) under sterile conditions and following nursing procedure in the following conditions:

        a. An emergency situation where it is determined that the trach is occluded and patient is in distress.

  b. When the trach cuff is leaking and the ventilator patient is unable to maintain tidal volume.

*Infection Control*

22. No large reservoir room humidifiers are allowed because of possibility of contamination.

23. Use new sterile suction set-ups with each suction attempt.

24. After suctioning, fold the catheter into the discarded glove to decrease cross contamination.

25. Change resuscitation bags q̄ 24 hours (by respiratory therapy).

26. Change solution bottles q̄ shift.

27. Change wall suction disposable containers q̄ shift along with tubing.

*Assessment*

28. Perform nursing assessment at least q̄ 4 hours with artificial airway patients in the following areas:

  a. Effective function of the airway in terms of patency and promoting effective ventilation

  b. Condition of mouth, nose, wound.

  c. Quantity and character (color, odor, consistency) of secretions

  d. Respiratory rate, character of respirations, temperature, and bilateral breath sounds.

  e. In addition, the chest is to be auscultated after all pulmonary/tube care and patient activity to determine correct placement of ET tube and possible movement into the right mainstem bronchus.

*Documentation*

29. Document the implementation: If the "Respiratory Protocol" on the Standards Flowsheet; an evaluative statement will be recorded in the shift narrative summary (or SOAP note) at the end of the shift in the Nurses Progress Record relative to patient physiologic and psychologic response to artificial airway.

*REFERENCES:*
*APPROVAL:*
*REVIEW:*
*REIVISION:*
*DISTRIBUTION:*

# FORMS/GUIDELINES

## INDEX

(Alphabetized by Name of form/Tool)

A 1. Anticoagulant Sheet      M

B      N

C      O

D      P

E      Q

F      R

G      S

H      T

I      U

J      V

K      W

L      X

     Y

     Z

# HOSPITAL
## DEPARTMENT OF NURSING

## GUIDELINES FOR ANTICOAGULANT FLOWSHEET

*PURPOSE:* To outline the proper use of the anticoagulant flowsheet in the recording of anticoagulant therapy and associated lab work.

*NATURE OF FORM:* The anticoagulant flow sheet is a permanent part of the record. It is a two-sided form completed in blue, black, or blue-black ink, and addressographed in the upper right hand corner.

*OPERATIONAL DEFINITIONS:*

*Anticoagulation*—the continuous or intermittant administration of medications designed to alter the clotting mechanism and thus prevent complications of thrombus formation and subsequent embolization.

*Pro-time*— a test of clotting time made by determining the time for clotting to occur after thromboplastin and calcium are added to decalcified plasma. This test is used primarily to evaluate the effectiveness of Coumadin.

*Partial thromboplastin time*—the clotting time of recalcified plasma in the presence of a lipid partial thromboplastin rather than complete thromboplastin of the prothrombin time test. Used to evaluate the effectiveness of Heparain therapy.

*PATIENT POPULATION:* This flowsheet is to be used on *every* patient placed on anticoagulant therapy regardless of the duration of treatment.

*RESPONSIBLE PERSONS*

1. The form will be pulled from the file, addressographed, and placed in the patient's record by the unit secretary on duty at the time the orders are noted for anticoagulant therapy.

2. Licensed nursing staff are responsible for recording on the form beginning with the initial lab values and/or medication administration.

3. All lab results for protimes and PTT's will be entered on this flowsheet at the time they are received by the lab, either by phone or by chart slip. This may be done by the unit secretary or licensed nurse.

4. All heparin and coumadin will be recorded on this flowsheet, including all loading doses, intermittant doses, and continuous infusions.

5. The unit secretary will discontinue the form when physicians orders are noted for stopping anticoagulation therapy.

*PLACEMENT IN CHART:* The form is placed in the patient's chart under the flow sheet section where it will be accessible to staff for medication documentation.

*INSTRUCTIONS:*

1. The form consists of three sections: one for lab results, one for anticoagulants administered, and one for signature validation.

2. The unit secretary will place intermittant coumadin and heparin on the patient's Medication Administration Record (MAR) for the purpose of unit dose replacement by pharmacy. However, the nurse may indicate that actual medication administration is recorded on the Anticoagulant Flowsheet. This will prevent duplication of charting. One time loading doses and continuous infusions will be entered on the kardex and recorded on this flowsheet by the responsible licensed nurse.

3. *LAB RESULTS*

   a. The responsible unit secretary or licensed nurse will enter lab results in proper column under "Prothromb. Time" or "Par. Thromb. Time". The former is used to evaluate Coumadin therapy and the latter used to evaluate Heparin therapy. The date and time of the result is entered. Two values are recorded: patient time and control time. Since all results are in seconds, this is assumed and need not be written.

   b. Initials of the reporting person are entered in the last column. These initials should be validated by full signature at the bottom of the record.

| Initials | Signature |
|----------|-----------|
| CSM | Carolyn Smith Marker, RN |

| ANTICOAGULANT FLOW SHEET | | | | | | | |
| --- | --- | --- | --- | --- | --- | --- | --- |
| LAB RESULTS | | | | | | | |
| | | COUMADIN | | HEPARIN | | | |
| DATE | TIME | PROTHROMB. TIME P.T. | | PAR. THROMB. TIME P.T.T. | | | INI. |
| | | PATIENT | CONT. | PATIENT | CONT. | | |
| 8/7/8 | 10 AM | 40 | 43 | | | | CSM |
| | | | | | | | |
| | | | | | | | |
| | | | | | | | |
| | | | | | | | |

4. *MEDICATION RECORD*

   a. The licensed nurse administering anticoagulants will record the dosage of Coumadin or Heparin in the proper column. The date and time of administration should accompany the dosage. These medications do not have to be duplicated on the MAR.

   b. Note that the Heparin column allows for recording of both intermittent doses of Heparin and continuous infusions. A notation should be made to indicate that the dose is a loading dose. Individual doses are recorded in the "Interm." column.

   c. Dosage levels of continuous infusion Heparin should be entered when the infusion is started, when lab values (PTT) are recorded, and whenever the physician orders a change in the units/hour. Continuous infusion rates are recorded in the column marked "CONT.".

   d. The licensed nurse completing the medication dosage column should enter his/her initials in the appropriate column and the identification signature at the bottom of the form.

   e. The comments section can be used to note loading dose, infusion started, rate of infusion increased or decreased, or therapy discontinued.

| Initials | Signature |
|---|---|
| JMK | Jacqueline M. Katz, RN |
| | |

## MEDICATION RECORD

| DATE | TIME | MEDICATION DOSAGE | | | INI. | COMMENTS |
|---|---|---|---|---|---|---|
| | | COUMADIN | HEPARIN | | | |
| | | | INTERM | CONT. | | |
| 3/26/8 | 11³⁰ am | mg | 5000 loading dose | u/hr | JMK | cont. infusion started |
| | 4pm | mg | 800 u | u/hr | JMK | ↑ infusion rate |
| | | mg | u | u/hr | | |
| | | mg | u | u/hr | | |
| | | mg | u | u/hr | | |

5. Note that all entries of anticoagulants are entered without skipping spaces. It may be necessary to skip spaces on the lab results column because every attempt should be made to have the lab values correlate with the current date and time of medication administration.

6. When discountinuing anticoagulant therapy, the comments section should indicate that this has been done along with the date, time, and signature of responsible licensed nurse.

7. See next page for completed example.

APPROVAL:
REVIEW:
REVISION:
DISTRIBUTION:

ADDRESSOGRAPH

LAB RESULTS
COUMADIN        HEPARIN

MEDICATION RECORD

| DATE | TIME | PROTHROMB. TIME P.T. PATIENT | PROTHROMB. TIME P.T. CONT. | PAR. THROMB. TIME P.T.T. PATIENT | PAR. THROMB. TIME P.T.T. CONT. | INI. | DATE | TIME | COUMADIN | HEPARIN INTERM | HEPARIN CONT. | INI. | COMMENTS |
|---|---|---|---|---|---|---|---|---|---|---|---|---|---|
| 9/1/81 | 8AM | | | 40 | 43 | PB | 9/1/81 | 10³⁰AM | mg | 5000 SQ u | u/hr | PB | |
| 9/1/81 | 9PM | | | 48 | 40 | MB | 9/1/81 | 4PM | mg | 5000 SQ u | u/hr | MB | |
| | | | | | | | 9/1/81 | 10PM | mg | 5000 SQ u | u/hr | MB | |
| | | | | | | | 9/2/81 | 4AM | mg | 5000 SQ u | u/hr | ML | |
| 9/2/81 | 9AM | | | 50 | 40 | JJ | 9/2/81 | 10AM | mg | u | 900 u/hr | SS | CONT. INFUSION STARTED |
| 9/2/81 | 2PM | | | 55 | 42 | JJ | 9/2/81 | 2PM | mg | u | 1200 u/hr | SS | ↑ INFUSION |
| 9/2/81 | 6PM | | | 59 | 40 | BJ | 9/2/81 | 6PM | mg | u | 1200 u/hr | BJ | INFUSION SAME |
| 9/3/81 | 10AM | | | 58 | 40 | PB | 9/3/81 | 10AM | mg | u | 1200 u/hr | PB | INFUSION RATE SAME |
| 9/4/81 | 10AM | | | 59 | 43 | PB | 9/4/81 | 10AM | mg | u | 1200 u/hr | PB | " |
| 9/5/81 | 10AM | 12 | 13 | 58 | 40 | PB | 9/5/81 | 10³⁰AM | 5 mg | u | 1200 u/hr | PB | STARTED ON COUMADIN |
| 9/6/81 | 12N | 18 | 12 | 62 | 40 | PB | 9/6/81 | 12³⁰P | 5 mg | u | 1200 u/hr | PB | |
| 9/7/81 | 10AM | 20 | 12 | 60 | 39 | PB | 9/7/81 | 10³⁰/A | 2.5 mg | u | u/hr | PB | CONT INFUSION DC'd |
| 9/8/81 | 10AM | 23 | 13 | | | JJ | 9/8/81 | 10³⁰/A | 2.5 mg | u | u/hr | JJ | C 16³⁰AM 9/7/81 |
| | | | | | | JJ | 9/8/81 | 10PM | 2.5 mg | u | u/hr | JJ | PB |
| 9/9/81 | 10AM | 26 | 12 | | | ML | 9/9/81 | 10PM | 2.0 mg | u | u/hr | ML | |
| | | | | | | | | | mg | u | u/hr | | |
| | | | | | | | | | mg | u | u/hr | | |
| | | | | | | | | | mg | u | u/hr | | |
| | | | | | | | | | mg | u | u/hr | | |
| | | | | | | | | | mg | u | u/hr | | |
| | | | | | | | | | mg | u | u/hr | | |

| Initials | Signature | Initials | Signature | Initials | Signature |
|---|---|---|---|---|---|
| PB | Peggy Brown, RN | ML | Mary Long, RN | | |
| MB | Margie Bower, RN | | | | |
| JJ | John Job, RN | | | | |
| BJ | Bonnie Jay, RN | | | | |
| | | | | | |

**DEPARTMENT OF NURSING**

*ANTICOAGULANT FLOW SHEET*

ADDRESSOGRAPH

*LAB RESULTS*
COUMADIN          HEPARIN

*MEDICATION RECORD*

| DATE | TIME | PROTHROMB. TIME P.T. | | PAR. THROMB. TIME P.T.T. | | INI. | DATE | TIME | MEDICATION DOSAGE | | | INI. | COMMENTS |
|------|------|--------|-------|---------|-------|------|------|------|----------|--------|--------|------|----------|
| | | PATIENT | CONT. | PATIENT | CONT. | | | | COUMADIN | HEPARIN INTERM | CONT. | | |
| | | | | | | | | | mg | u | u/hr | | |
| | | | | | | | | | mg | u | u/hr | | |
| | | | | | | | | | mg | u | u/hr | | |
| | | | | | | | | | mg | u | u/hr | | |
| | | | | | | | | | mg | u | u/hr | | |
| | | | | | | | | | mg | u | u/hr | | |
| | | | | | | | | | mg | u | u/hr | | |
| | | | | | | | | | mg | u | u/hr | | |
| | | | | | | | | | mg | u | u/hr | | |
| | | | | | | | | | mg | u | u/hr | | |
| | | | | | | | | | mg | u | u/hr | | |
| | | | | | | | | | mg | u | u/hr | | |
| | | | | | | | | | mg | u | u/hr | | |
| | | | | | | | | | mg | u | u/hr | | |
| | | | | | | | | | mg | u | u/hr | | |
| | | | | | | | | | mg | u | u/hr | | |
| | | | | | | | | | mg | u | u/hr | | |
| | | | | | | | | | mg | u | u/hr | | |
| | | | | | | | | | mg | u | u/hr | | |
| | | | | | | | | | mg | u | u/hr | | |

| Initials | Signature | | Initials | Signature | | Initials | Signature | |
|----------|-----------|--|----------|-----------|--|----------|-----------|--|
| | | | | | | | | |
| | | | | | | | | |
| | | | | | | | | |
| | | | | | | | | |
| | | | | | | | | |

**HOSPITAL**

**DEPARTMENT OF NURSING**

<table>
<tr><td colspan="2">INITIATED</td><td colspan="2">DISCONTINUED</td></tr>
<tr><td colspan="2">DATE _____</td><td colspan="2">DATE _____</td></tr>
<tr><td colspan="2">TIME _____</td><td colspan="2">TIME _____</td></tr>
<tr><td colspan="2">RN _____</td><td colspan="2">RN _____</td></tr>
</table>

STANDARD OF CARE (SCP-three column)
ON PATIENTS WITH: *CHF*

| INITIATED | | NURSING DIAGNOSIS | PATIENT OUTCOMES | EVALUATED | | NURSING INTERVENTIONS | RESOLVED | |
| DATE | RN | PATIENT CARE PROBLEM | | DATE | RN | | DATE | RN |
|---|---|---|---|---|---|---|---|---|
| | | 1. Altered cardiac output (CO) related to inadequate inotropic activity. | Patient will maintain sufficient CO to support functional body systems. | | | 1. Assess body systems for objective evidence of progressive CHF each shift to include the following:<br><br>• Apical/radial pulse for one minute for rate/regularity.<br>• Neck veins c̄ 45° for ↑JVP.<br>• B/P (position of comfort).<br>• Respiratory rate and character (degree of effort, use of accessory muscles, orthopnea, pillows required).<br>• Posterior chest auscultation for rales/rhonchi/wheezing (inspir./expir.).<br>• Abdomen for distention, BS., RUQ discomfort.<br>• Lower extremities (hands and dependent body parts) for presence and degree of edema (1, 2, 3 plus).<br>• Presence of calf tenderness.<br><br>2. Carry out subjective assessment each shift. Include the following:<br><br>• Excessive fatigue, • Palpatations,<br>• Dyspnea (new or ↑), • Nausea,<br>• PND/insomnia, • Dizziness,<br>• Light headedness, • Chest pain<br><br>3. Record findings every shift on assessment flowsheet per guidelines.<br><br>4. Report following findings to MD within 15 minutes as evidence of exaggerated LVF:<br><br>*(continue to next page)* | | |

| INITIATED | | NURSING DIAGNOSIS | PATIENT OUTCOMES | EVALUATED | | NURSING INTERVENTIONS | RESOLVED | |
|---|---|---|---|---|---|---|---|---|
| DATE | RN | PATIENT CARE PROBLEM | | DATE | RN | | DATE | RN |
| | | | | | | • respiratory rate > 26/minute,<br>• altered LOC/mental confusion,<br>• excessive dyspnea (rest or activity),<br>• persistent cough/PND/orthopnea,<br>• significant color change or sweating,<br>• chest pain,<br>• greater chest congestion,<br>• HR>110 or <55 BPM,<br>• new rhythm irregularity or worsening of known arrhythmia; be especially alert to the establishment of a *regular* rhythm in a patient with known atrial fibrillation on digitalis.<br><br>5. Apply 0₂ at L/minute via cannula along with bed/chair rest; implement *Chest Pain Protocol* and *12 Lead EKG Protocol* as indicated; perform full physical assessment; stay with patient.<br><br>6. If patient condition does not improve within 15 minutes, notify MD.<br><br>7. Record all observations/ interventions on Standards NFS and NPR. | | |
| | | 2. Potential alteration in fluid balance related to volume overload or excessive diuresis. | Patient will achieve and maintain an adequate circulating volume. | | | 1. Weigh patient daily and record on I/O record; report gain >2lbs/24 hours).<br><br>2. Report positive fluid balance (>1 liter/24 hours).<br><br>3. Place on I/O every 8 hours if positive fluid balance is evident; if UO less than sufficient; if 3+ edema develops; if pulmonary edema develops.<br><br>4. Place on I/O if on IV's (use only microdrips and 500cc bottles; all IV's to be on IVAC's).<br><br>5. Discuss with MD the ordering of electrolytes every 48 hours if patient is newly placed on diuretics.<br><br>6. Discuss with MD the ordering of electrolytes if patient urinary output >2000cc/24 hours or 1000cc/shift.<br><br>7. If patient on diuretics, perform specific gravity on urine qod; if urine concentrated, skin turgor poor, or mucous membranes dry, discuss fluid volume replacement with MD.<br><br>*(continued on next page)* | | |

| INITIATED | | NURSING DIAGNOSIS | PATIENT OUTCOMES | EVALUATED | | NURSING INTERVENTIONS | RESOLVED | |
|---|---|---|---|---|---|---|---|---|
| DATE | RN | PATIENT CARE PROBLEM | | DATE | RN | | DATE | RN |
| | | 3. Potential activity intolerance. | The patient will balance energy demands to his current capabilities. | | | 1. Determine patients energy capability through observation and assessment of physical response to ADL and nursing care; alter activity and rest periods accordingly. | | |
| | | | | | | 2. Place at rest for 30-60 minutes after meals. | | |
| | | | | | | 3. Follow activity level ordered by MD with full explanation of limitations to patient; record patients response to activity levels q̄ shift on progressive activity record per guidelines. | | |
| | | | | | | 4. Maintain semi-fowler's while in bed unless high requested by patient. | | |
| | | | | | | 5. If "Progressive Activity Protocol" ordered by MD, implement schedule, evaluating patient response and documenting activities as directed. | | |
| | | 4. Need for accurate pharmacologic intervention. | Patient will achieve maximum benefit from physician ordered meds through appropriate nursing intervention. | | | 1. Administer all medications within 15 minutes of due time and document effects with an evaluation statement in NPR each shift; observe for orthostatic hypotension after every major position change. | | |
| | | | | | | 2. Review name/dosage/purpose/side effects with patient/SO at administration time of all p.o. cardiac meds and Nitroglycerin paste. | | |
| | | | | | | 3. Clarify with physician whether patient to be on self medication program; identify "home" drugs 48 hours prior to discharge and begin "Cardiac Drug Instruction Protocol". | | |
| | | | | | | 4. Integrate appropriate drug protocols into nursing routines: (circle current ones in effect):<br>• Nitroglycerin Protocol,<br>• Antiarrhythmic Protocol,<br>• Inotropic Drug Protocol. | | |

(continued on next page)

| INITIATED | | NURSING DIAGNOSIS / PATIENT CARE PROBLEM | PATIENT OUTCOMES | EVALUATED | | NURSING INTERVENTIONS | RESOLVED | |
|---|---|---|---|---|---|---|---|---|
| DATE | RN | | | DATE | RN | | DATE | RN |
| | | 5. Potential for acute LVF (pulmonary edema). | Patient will be free of potential lethal effects of extreme pulmonary congestion. | | | 1. Assess patient each shift for evidence of pulmonary edema as indicated by: <br><br> • extreme SOB/coughing, <br> • HR> 120/minute, <br> • frothy sputum, <br> • extensive rales/rhonchi/wheezing, <br> • agitation/cyanosis. <br><br> 2. If evident, implement the following actions: (STAY WITH PATIENT!!) <br><br> • Notify MD immediately; <br> • Perform quick baseline assessment with emphasis on respiratory, tissue perfusion, neuro, status to estimate degree of threat to life, check full V/S; <br> • Position patient in high-fowler's in bed or chair (chair preferable) if B/P allows; <br> • Start $O_2$ at 6/L. via MASK; <br> • Start IV of 500cc $D_5W$ with catheter KVO (25cc/hour); <br> • Perform stat EKG, noting life threatening PVB's; <br> • Order stat chest xray, requesting wet reading; <br> • Have crash cart in readiness; <br><br> 3. Record all assessment/interventions in NPR; enter verbal order for EKG and chest xray on order sheet; MD to sign with in 24 hrs. | | |
| | | 6. Potential anxiety/fear related to symptoms and prognosis. | Patient/SO will express concern appropriate for condition and avoid excessive fearfulness. | | | 1. Assess anxiety level each shift of patient and SO; identify usual coping mechanisms to acute and chronic stress. <br><br> 2. Encourage patient/SO to express concerns and respond accordingly documenting these for followup by other staff. <br><br> 3. Provide full explanations for all medical and nursing therapies; encourage self care activities as physical state allows especially in area of ADL, self medication, and progressive activity monitoring. | | |
| | | 7. Potential knowledge deficit for self care. | Patient/SO will perform self care as identified in CHF Teaching Protocol. | | | 1. Determine patient/SO current understanding of CHF pathology, symptomatology, activity/diet restrictions, and medication regimens. <br><br> 2. Implement *CHF Teaching Protocol* within 48 hours prior to discharge. <br><br> 3. Record patient response on protocol as directed. | | |

REFERENCES:
APPROVAL:
REVIEW:
REVISION:
DISTRIBUTION:

<table>
<tr><td colspan="2">

**HOSPITAL**
**DEPARTMENT OF NURSING**

</td><td>

| INITIATED |
DATE _____
TIME _____
RN _____

</td><td>

| DISCONTINUED |
DATE _____
TIME _____
RN _____

</td></tr>
</table>

STANDARD OF CARE (SCS) ON
PATIENTS WITH: *Inguinal Herniorrhaphy (overnight stay)*

| OUTCOME STANDARDS: | DATE MET/SIGN |
|---|---|
| PHYSIOLOGIC: ▶ Patient will achieve a stable, comfortable post op state without complications or infection. | |
| PYSCHOLOGIC: ▶ Patient will express acceptance of limitations of activity imposed by surgical correction. | |
| COGNITIVE: ▶ Patient will explain essential components of self care for discharge. | |

| INITIATED | | SUBJECT HEADINGS | NURSING INTERVENTIONS | DISCONTINUED | |
| DATE | RN | | | DATE | RN |
|---|---|---|---|---|---|
| | | 1. Inadequate preparation for the OR related to physiologic status, knowledge base, and anxiety level. | 1. Implement *Pre-Op Management Protocol* (checklist).<br>2. Implement *Pre-Op Teaching Protocol* and document on tool patient's response.<br>3. Complete short stay NDB. | | |
| | | 2. Altered physiologic status related to post op condition. | 1. Implement *Post Op Protocol.*<br>2. Document protocol implementation each shift on Standards NFS.<br>3. Document patient response to post op care in NPR each shift with specific emphasis on:<br>　　▲ adequacy of respiratory status,<br>　　▲ nutritional and elimination status,<br>　　▲ progressive ambulation ability. | | |
| | | 3. Pain related to surgical manipulation + muscle spasm. | 1. Monitor incisional pain by direct questioning at 2-4 hour intervals q̄ shift; encourage patient to notify staff of discomfort early.<br>2. Instruct patient to use side position with affected leg flexed slightly to reduce muscle strain and keep similar position flexion when on back.<br>3. Support affected leg with small folded bath blanket. Avoid pressure to impede circulation.<br>4. Specifically assess scrotal swelling/pain; if present apply ice pack as patient desires.<br>5. Use ordered analgesics as needed, progressing patient to PO meds *within 6-12 hours.*<br>6. Record pain med/response in NFS/MAR within *20 minutes* of action. | | |

| STANDARD OF CARE (SCS) ON PATIENTS WITH: *Inguinal Herniorrhaphy (overnight stay)* (continued) | | | | | |
|---|---|---|---|---|---|
| INITIATED | | SUBJECT HEADINGS | NURSING INTERVENTIONS | DISCONTINUED | |
| DATE | RN | | | DATE | RN |
| | | 4. Potential for wound infection. | 1. Leave initial surgical dressing intact until changed by MD (usually early AM prior to disch.)<br>2. Change dressing only if unduly soiled or excessive drainage present—report latter to MD.<br>3. Instruct patient on:<br>▲ proper handwashing,<br>▲ dressing routine change 2nd P.O day,<br>▲ leaving wound open to air after that,<br>▲ S/S of swelling, redress, drainage, excessive pain to report to MD. | | |
| | | 5. Potential for bowel involvement. | 1. Read MD operative note as part of initial post op care to be aware of degree of this problem.<br>2. Auscultate for early appropriate return of bowel sounds.<br>3. Assess for unusual or excessive abdominal pain.<br>4. Report abnormal BS or abd. pain to surgeon promptly. | | |
| | | 6. Potential for anxiety related to knowledge deficit for self care. | 1. Assess patient/SO current understanding of hernia pathology & surgical correction.<br>2. Review following items:<br>▲ wound care,<br>▲ signs/symptoms to report,<br>▲ comfort measures and pain management.<br>3. Provide/review post op physician instruction sheet with emphasis on limited exercise, avoidance of strenuous activity or lifting until approved by MD.<br>4. Elicit questions.<br>5. Document patient's response and meeting of discharge criteria on Discharge Form.<br>6. Complete and record in ᴎᴦR final discharge assessment (per unit routine).<br>7 Indicate positive outcome standards in Standard of Care. | | |

*REFERENCES:*
*APPROVAL:*
*REVIEW:*
*REVISION:*
*DISTRIBUTION:*

# GLOSSARY

**ADDENDUM**—one or more typed pages that address additional policy content; deals with very specific, detailed, changable information; is labeled with a title and an alphabetical designation; is referred to in the main body of structure and arranged alphabetically behind a set of structure standards.

**APPROVAL (Mechanism)**— refers to the serial activities, dates, and persons or groups of persons used to give a standard official sanction; provides the legitimacy, credibility, and clout needed to successfully implement a standard; listed at the bottom of a standard (or alternate location) and includes both the date and mechanism.

**COMPONENTS**— refers to a content item in a process standard; for example a procedure consists of nine components including Title, Purpose, Supportive Data, Equipment List, Content, Documentation, Reference, Approval/Review/Revision, and Distribution.

**DEPARTMENT**— refers commonly to an organized subdivision of a total health care system, as in Department of Nursing.

**DEPENDENT**— refers to nursing actions which are delegated from the medical staff and require physicians orders prior to implementation.

**DEPENDENT PROTOCOL**— a nursing protocol that outlines patient care measures of a dependent nature; usually deals with diagnostic and therapeutic interventions that are reimbursable by third party payors such as x-rays, lab tests, drug therapies, and electrical therapies.

**DIVISION**— refers commonly to a cluster of nursing units that are similar in patient population, staffing, and environment.

**DRAFTING FORM**— one or several sheets of pre-typed paper that demonstrates the writing style of a format of a process standard, such as a drafting form for a procedure or protocol; assists staff to outline content quickly.

**ELEMENT**— refers to specifically identified aspects of structure; consists of 13 items in generic Department of Nursing Structure Standards and 9 items in Unit Specific Structure Standards.

**FORMAT**— refers to the various forms in which a process standard may be written; there are six formats of process standards including job description, performance standards, procedures, protocols, guidelines, and standards of care.

**GENERIC**— applicable across the entire Department of Nursing.

**GENERIC STRUCTURE STANDARDS**— the set of policies outlining the operation of a Department of Nursing covering 13 elements of structure.

**GC...**— the format ic writing an outcome standard which may be in the style of a nursing goa. or a patient outcome.

**GOVERNING RULE**— one of the essential elements of both generic and unit specific structure standards that deals with such items of content as infection control, equipment, preventive maintenance, or safety; there are 16 content items at the generic level and 8 at the unit level.

**GROUP**— a predefined patient population; consistent with diagnostic category, admitting or discharge diagnosis, medical diagnosis, or DRG (diagnosis related group).

**GUIDELINES**— a format of a process standard which outlines how to complete and use a nursing tool or form for communication or documentation.

**HIERARCHY**— a graded arrangement of items; in relation to standards, the hierarchy means that the structure standards form a foundation of practice; process standards then are addressed next to define staff performance and patient care; outcome standards are addressed last to specify end results and constitute the apex of the Marker Model.

**INDEPENDENT**— refers to nursing actions that are capable of being implemented by nursing without direction or permission by the medical staff.

**INDEPENDENT PROTOCOL**— a nursing protocol that outlines patient care measures of an independent nature; may be carried out by the nursing staff by nursing order only, without requiring physician order.

**INTERDEPENDENT**— refers to nursing actions that are mixed, some being independent and some dependent.

**INTERDEPENDENT PROTOCOL**— a nursing protocol that is mixed and outlines patient care measures of both a dependent and independent nature; requires a physician's order for the dependent functions prior to implementation.

**JOB DESCRIPTION**— the first format of process standards; a brief overview of duties, responsibilities, and qualifications for a level of worker.

**KEY WORDS**— one or two word terms chosen to organize nursing care content around in nursing protocols.

**LEVEL OF EMPLOYEE**— refers to a category of worker who is hired to do a certain job outlined in a job description because he/she meets the qualifications.

**LEVEL OF STRUCTURE**— refers to the level at which structure standards are written; may be generic and directed at the department or unit specific and directed at a particular nursing unit.

**MARKER MODEL**— a comprehensive and systematic method for defining professional nursing practice in terms of systems operation, staff performance and patient care, and results.

**NURSING GOAL**— a style of writing an outcome standard which begins with an action verb, is directed at the nursing staff, and identifies a desired nursing result.

**NURSING INTERVENTION**— a series of actions (both dependent and independent) written as part of a protocol or standard of care to direct the staff in what is to be implemented as nursing care; specifically identifies one of the columns in a standard of care (both SCP's and SCS's).

**OBJECTIVES**— one of the elements of structure standards at both the generic and unit specific levels; specifies what a Department of Nursing, Division, or Unit is trying to accomplish during a designated time period; may be written to define ongoing aspirations and be of a permanent nature; or may be written to define short-term (weeks to several months) project accomplishments in a nursing area (ie. Management by Objectives).

**OUTCOME**— a result of care given.

**OUTCOME STANDARDS**— a type of standard that defines results; written in the format of goals.

**PATIENT OUTCOMES**— a style of writing an outcome standard which begins with "The Patient will . . . ", is directed at the patient, and identifies a desired physiologic, psychologic, or cognitive state to be achieved.

**PERFORMANCE STANDARDS**— a series of statements which outline the expectations of a group of nurses; extension of the job description that delineates required behaviors that are both specific and measurable; directed toward a patient population, acuity levels, and leadership values; the second format of a process standard.

**POLICY**— the format for writing structure standards; written as a set following a combination outline and paragraph style; covers defined elements of structure; generally limited to approximately 60 pages for a Department of Nursing and 15 pages for a Nursing Unit.

**PROCEDURE**— the third format of a process standard; outlines how to perform a psychomotor skill; has a technical and theoretical basis.

**PROCESS**— a type of standard (process standard) that defines actions and behaviors required of staff in carrying out care as well as what constitutes that care; process standards are directed at the nurse or the patient.

**PROTOCOL**— the fourth format of a process standard; defines the care and management of a broad patient care problem or issue in 5 categories: non-invasive and invasive equipment; diagnostic, prophylactic, and therapeutic measures; physiologic and psychologic states; and nursing diagnosis.

**QUALITY ASSURANCE**— a process in which standards are set and action is taken to insure compliance to the standards; predefined activities that are designed, implemented, and documented to demonstrate compliance to established standards.

**REVIEW**— refers to the date that appears at the bottom (or alternate location) of a standard indicating when the standard is due for review.

**REVISION—** refers to the date that appears at the bottom (or alternate location) of a standard indicating when the standard was last reviewed for currency and appropriateness.

**STANDARD—** written statements defining a level of practice in the staff or a set of conditions in the patient or staff determined to be acceptable by some authority.

**STANDARD OF CARE—** the sixth format of a process standard; defining the prewritten care for a group of patients with common problems.

**STANDARD CARE PLAN—** a style of a standard of care (process standard) which outlines the care of a particular patient population (DRG); generally limited to 2 pages (back and front) and formally designed into 2, 3, or 4 columns; identifies priority nursing diagnosis/patient care problems, patient outcomes, and nursing interventions for a group of patients.

**STANDARD CARE STATEMENT—** an alternate style of a standard of care (process standard) which outlines the care of a particular patient population (DRG); generally limited to 2 pages (back and front); organizes information simply under "Subject Heading" and "Nursing Intervention"; less formal and sophisticated than SCP's; often used to define care for patient populations in short stay/rapid turnover nursing areas.

**STANDARDS MANUAL—** the primary reference tool in a Department of Nursing and Nursing Unit that houses and organizes all written nursing standards; may be generic for the Department of Nursing or specific for a particular nursing unit.

**STRUCTURE—** a type of standard that outlines the conditions and mechanisms needed to give patient care; directed at the system and defines the operation of that system.

**STYLE—** refers to the technical manner in which a specific format of standard is written; for example, an outcome standard is written as a goal; that goal may be written in the style of a nursing goal or a patient outcome.

**TEACHING PROTOCOL—** a specific style of protocol designed especially to outline nursing responsibilities in patient education; defines the desired patient outcomes, content to be taught, the teaching methods, and documents these activities as well as patient response.

**TYPE—** refers to a kind of standard. There are three—structure, process, outcome.

**UNIT—** refers to a circumscribed, geographical area providing care to a defined patient population by a permanently assigned staff.

**UNIT SPECIFIC—** refers to standards which are written for a specified unit and are applicable to that unit (or group of units) only.